EPILEPSY INFORMATION
A PATIENT FRIENDLY
RESOURCE FOR SEIZURES

SECOND EDITION

8/14

ISBN-10: 1494224437
ISBN-13: 9781494224431

Visit www.createspace.com/1000250976 to order additional copies.

EPILEPSY INFORMATION
A PATIENT FRIENDLY
RESOURCE FOR SEIZURES

SECOND EDITION

by

Diane M. Keeler

EPILEPSY INFORMATION
A PATIENT FRIENDLY RESOURCE
FOR SEIZURES

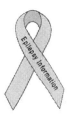

There's no more, *"I don't understand"* because of all the big medical words. No more undesired information. This book is easy to read and understand as it's presented to you in a simplistic refreshing way. All medical terminology is explained directly with the text or can be found in the glossary.

You'll learn how to deal with all the many issues that directly affect your daily life. The information enclosed can help make your life much more tolerable and much more knowledgeable. If you want to gain better control over your life, this book is for you!

This book is:

- *Edited by an epileptologist for medical accuracy.*

- *Updated regularly to provide new information when released and confirmed.*

Used books may not be the most recent version.

Disclaimer: I do not imply or express any guarantee or responsibility with respect to any information and recommendations provided inside this book. This book is not a substitute for a medical professional's advice! It's designed for supplemental reasons only.

A SPECIAL THANK YOU

Jesus Christ, *My Lord and Savior* for strengthening me spiritually, physically, emotionally, and for making me stronger and complete. For giving me the physical ability and compassion to be an epilepsy advocate. *He is the Way, the Truth, and the Life,* John 14:6

Kim, *Husband and best friend,* for loving me unconditionally during my battle with epilepsy. For picking me up when I was down, literally and physically. For supporting me and helping to make it easier for me to be the epilepsy advocate I long to be.

John S. Freeman, *Cover designer, photographer, "photoshopper;" and friend* for leading me to the right doctor and freely offering the many specialties in which he perfects. Without his help, this book would not have lived up to my expectations.

Joyce D. Liporace M.D. *Director of Women's Health and Epilepsy Program, Neurologist, and Epileptologist,* for her sincere commitment and concern for all epilepsy patients through both treatment and education. I'm thankful that she doesn't just treat the condition but the person as a whole. Her professionalism has lead me into an improved seizure controlled life. And far from least, she taught me priceless information in which I'm now able to pass on through this book.

Michael R. Sperling M.D., *Baldwin Keyes Professor of Neurology at Thomas Jefferson University Hospital and Director of Jefferson Comprehensive Epilepsy Center,* for his unending effort and perseverance in expanding and managing research in order to achieve advancement of medical treatment for epilepsy patients everywhere.

Michael J. O'Connor M.D., *Neurologist, Neurophysiologist, Epileptologist*, for his genuine care for epilepsy patients and continuous dedication in broadening education.

William M. O'Connor, and James J. Evans Neurosurgeons, for their professionalism, compassion, and expertise in removing troublesome brain tissue and giving me one of the greatest gifts anyone can give, a new chance at life.

Thomas Jefferson University Hospital Nurses and Certified Nursing Assistants, for professionally and compassionately caring for me. No words can truly express my appreciation for all they have given me.

Epilepsy Foundation for providing precious help to everyone in the epilepsy community.

Table of Contents

MEDICAL INFORMATION

APPENDIX

Interesting

Information

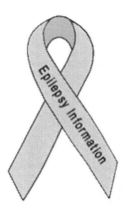

The History of Epilepsy

Learning the history of epilepsy is significant in order to appreciate how the world of epilepsy has advanced, especially concerning treatment techniques. After reading this chapter, you'll certainly agree that we are truly blessed to be living in modern times.

Epilepsy has always existed and has affected billions of people worldwide. It is one of the world's oldest known health conditions affecting the human race which until recent years was grossly misunderstood. The word epilepsy comes from a Greek word meaning, to possess, seize or hold. Through the ages, people with epilepsy were isolated from society sometimes through imprisonment, committed into insane institutions, exorcised, and tortured only because people believed they were witches or demon possessed. Depending on what part of the world the "witches" lived, they suffered a variety of torture techniques including but not exclusive to; burned alive at the stake, forced to consume heated or scalding consumables such as hot coal and boiling water, crushed to death, buried alive, dismembered, drowned by raising then dunking repeatedly until finally drowned.

People, who were believed to be demon possessed, were attempted to be cured by priests through magic and prayers. Most people with epilepsy were outcasts from society and punished frequently. But thankfully ancient physicians, Atreya of India and Hippocrates of Greece recognized seizures as a neurological dysfunction rather than a supernatural event therefore challenging the diagnosis of evil spirits. They recognized the cause of seizures was due to brain abnormalities not demonic powers. Unfortunately, the belief of demon possession continued throughout time. Negative attitudes continued even after proof that epilepsy was a health condition.

Today, the majority of people who lack information about epilepsy have a predisposition to compare it with insanity and mental retardation. As you know, this is simply not true! Many people with epilepsy have normal or above–average intelligence. Epilepsy is non discriminatory. It affects both men and women, of all ages and race.

Mysticism and Fear is the Ancestry of Epilepsy

Ancient Babylonians thought seizures were due to demons assaulting the person. Forty tablets exist from 2000 B.C. which actually records various types of seizures. Every seizure type was associated with the name of a god, and was considered a spiritual condition that was evil. The treatments used were of a spiritual nature.

Ancient Greeks believed epilepsy was due to offending the moon goddess, Selene. One of the cures was to eat mistletoe which was picked without using a blade or sickle during the time when the moon appeared to be smallest. The mistletoe could not touch the ground. They believed if it did, it would be ineffective against the "falling sickness," since it had fallen also.

Ancient Romans believed epilepsy came from demons and was contagious by touching someone with epilepsy or simply by being breathed on by them. People would spit to get rid of the demon. Since they considered epilepsy contagious, people with epilepsy had to live alone.

During the Middle Ages in Europe Epilepsy was identified as the "falling sickness." People looked to relics and saints for cures. Saint Valentine and the three wise men were predominantly important patrons of people with epilepsy. If you had epilepsy, you could receive a specially blessed ring that would help manage your seizure activity. This thinking was still around in colonial America. George Washington's step daughter was treated with an iron ring.

During the Renaissance Period People started examining ancient scripts again, which revitalized the past ideas. Some people believed that individuals with epilepsy were prophets! They thought they could see the past, present, and future through the seizure during their state of unconsciousness. The belief was that they were very intelligent based on some people who had epilepsy in the Roman Empire, including Julius Cesar! Regardless of the good that was considered an aspect of epilepsy, it continued to be seen as a dreadful disease by the average person.

1486, the handbook, Malleus Maleficarum Latin for "The Hammer of Witches," was written and was considered the most distinguished medieval manual on witches. It was first published in 1487 and was rapidly spread throughout Europe with the help of the newly created printing press. Its main objective was to teach judges how to recognize, cross-examine, and persecute witches. The handbook taught that one method to identify a witch was by the presence of seizures. It encouraged torture which caused the death of more than 200,000 women who were believed to be witches.

The late 1600's in Colonial America People with epilepsy were believed to be overtaken by demonic powers. Any woman who experienced seizures was a "handmaiden of the devil."

400 B.C. Hippocrates, known as the "Father of Medicine," wrote the first book on epilepsy titled, *On the Sacred Disease*. He made it clear that people do not get epilepsy from "the gods" because that would be considering gods as bad. He noted that even though epilepsy is "sacred" it appeared to him as no more divine or sacred than any other affliction. He blatantly remarks that men regarded its cause as divine due to their ignorance simply because it is dissimilar to other afflictions. He felt the notion of epilepsy's divinity was due to their inability to comprehend it! The spiritual cure during that period in time was to sleep in the temple overnight and have faith that the god, Asclepius would come forward in a dream and cure them or tell them how to acquire a cure.

It's safe to say, we are blessed to be living in modern times since epilepsy is now recognized as a medical condition. We now have the privilege to live without the fear that has gone before us in which we truly can't comprehend. And best of all, we now have treatment that is functional not spiritual!

Historical Facts

2,000 B.C. dates brain surgery for epilepsy treatment in the South American area! The surgical tools used at that time were made of hand-shaped obsidian (a hard volcanic rock with sharp edges) and bronze! Success rates were high! The patients experienced improved health.

19th Century Neurology was recognized different from a psychiatric condition. The theory of epilepsy as a brain disorder became more extensively accepted which helped to lessen the stigma connected with the disorder. People who had critical epilepsy in addition to psychiatric disorders were cared for in asylums. However, the two groups were kept divided since seizures were believed to be contagious.

1857 Bromide was the world's first effective antiepileptic medication. It was widely used in the United States and Europe.

1859-1906 The modern medical era of epilepsy began. It was then that a seizure was defined as; an excessive, occasional, and disorderly discharge of nerve tissue on muscles. And that seizure activity can change behavior, consciousness, and sensation.

Early 1900's Some U.S. states had laws forbidding people with epilepsy to marry or become parents, and some states permitted sterilization.

1904 The title "epileptologist" was used to identify a doctor who specializes in epilepsy. William Spratling was the first epileptologist in North America since he created the title.

1920's Females were restricted from having children. Many were forced to have hysterectomies to prevent pregnancy.

1920 The ketogenic diet was designed which effectively decreased or even cured some people from seizure activity. It is one of the oldest types of epilepsy treatments. There were few effective treatments for epilepsy up to that point.

1929 The electroencephalogram was a major breakthrough as it was announced to the world by German psychiatrist, Hans Berger as an accurate method to record electric currents in the brain without opening the skull as well as to provide details of seizure activity on a simple strip of paper!

1968 The Epilepsy Foundation of America now known as the Epilepsy Foundation was founded.

1997 The Food and Drug Administration (FDA) approved the vagus nerve stimulator for partial epilepsy, in combination with medication.

Theories, Comments, and Controversy

Epilepsy has occupied a great deal of awareness in the medical community, since the beginning of time! Barely any other medical condition has stimulated so much discussion and attracted so much attention as epilepsy. Aristotle was the first person known to suggest the connection of epilepsy and genius. Reflecting on the probability of genius and epilepsy brings many theories, comments, and controversy by neurology professors, neuropsychologists, and neurologists.

The most common controversy is; if damage happens to part of the brain while still developing, the corresponding brain on the other side has the opportunity to overdevelop. There is no evidence at this time regarding the connection with epilepsy and genius. However, there is evidence that epilepsy does *not* do the opposite.

Regardless of the theories, comments, and controversy, the record speaks for itself. See: *Famous People with Epilepsy*

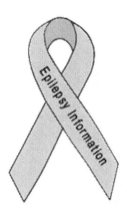

Myths and Facts

Even with medical proof in modern times, epilepsy is still viewed in ways which misrepresent the truth behind the neurological disorder causing a stigma which glazes over truth about epilepsy. Despite the great amount of people affected by epilepsy, it is still extremely misunderstood. It can be the source of many emotional and social problems for people like you and me. These powerful negative stereotypes can affect a person profoundly.

We all know what it's like to feel the prejudice from the uneducated public concerning epilepsy. In an effort to dispel all the ridiculous common misconceptions, the following myths and facts will prepare you to defend our condition respectfully.

The majority of the following myths won't make you happy but they will give you ammunition to fight back against the idiotic comments and beliefs people still have in the 21st century!

Myth: During a seizure, a person can swallow their tongue and suffocate.
Fact: It's physically impossible to swallow your tongue! If you don't believe me, all you have to do is touch the roof of your mouth with

the tip of your tongue. Feel the little flap of skin (frenulum) under your tongue. That flap is what keeps your tongue in place!

Myth: You should force something into the mouth of someone having a seizure.
Fact: Absolutely NOT!! That's a good way to break a jaw, chip teeth, puncture gums, and even suffocate the person you're trying to help.

Myth: Someone with epilepsy shouldn't use a computer for a long time.
Fact: The computer is no more dangerous to a person with epilepsy than a television. The only time either one is a threat is when it involves someone who has photosensitive seizures that are triggered by flashing lights.

Myth: You should restrain someone having a seizure.
Fact: Never use restraint! The seizure will run its course. You can never forcefully stop a seizure. That will be as successful as trying to forcefully stop someone from having the hiccups! Using restraint could seriously injure the person you're trying to help more than the seizure itself.

Myth: Epilepsy is contagious.
Fact: You cannot "catch" epilepsy from someone else. Epilepsy is a neurological condition and is as contagious as diabetes or cancer.

Myth: People with epilepsy are disabled and can't work.
Fact: People with epilepsy work just like the rest of society. Some people are more challenged to be a part of the work force but most are successfully productive in challenging careers. See: *Famous People with Epilepsy*

Myth: People with epilepsy shouldn't be in jobs of responsibility and stress.
Fact: Many people with epilepsy have effectively achieved stressful demanding careers that are both mentally and physically challenging such as; administration, government, and professional sports just to name a few. See: *Famous People with Epilepsy*

Myth: Epilepsy is rare and there aren't very many people who have it.
Fact: There are approximately 2.7 million people in the United States alone and 40 million worldwide. There are more than twice as many people with epilepsy in North America as the number of people with cerebral palsy, muscular dystrophy, multiple sclerosis, and cystic fibrosis *combined*.

Myth: Epilepsy starts from childhood.
Fact: Epilepsy can start at any age from birth to 100!

Myth: You can't tell what a person might do during a seizure.
Fact: Each type of seizure takes on common characteristics and each person's action will be the same during each episode.

Myth: People with epilepsy are physically limited in what they can do.
Fact: In most cases, epilepsy isn't a wall to physical achievement. However, there are some cases, where individuals are more severely affected due to the type and amount of seizures which may limit them.

Myth: Epilepsy is a psychological condition.
Fact: Epilepsy is a medical/neurological condition. Seizures are the result of an excessive and disorderly discharge of electrical energy in the brain. It is much like a thunderstorm within the skull.

Myth: If you have a seizure, you have epilepsy.
Fact: Seizures are a symptom of epilepsy. Having a single seizure or even several does not necessarily mean a person has epilepsy. Epilepsy means recurrent seizures.

Myth: People with epilepsy are in some way brain damaged, mentally ill, or retarded.
Fact: Even though epilepsy involves the brain doesn't mean the person is mentally affected. Epilepsy is a physical medical condition. Many people with epilepsy are extremely smart and gifted.

Myth: You can help a person "snap out" of a seizure.
Fact: It's not possible to stop someone from having a seizure. Therefore, there's no benefit in shaking, yelling or holding them down or any other type of aggressive approach. The best thing anyone can

do is keep them as safe and comfortable as possible. See: *Seizure Types and Triggers*

Myth: Epilepsy consists of grand mal seizures only.
Fact: Epilepsy has many forms ranging from violent convulsions to momentary lapses of attention. See: *Seizure Types and Triggers*

Myth: Most seizures are quick and not infrequent.
Fact: Seizure activity has variable aspects in every person. No one person is the same.

Myth: Epilepsy spirals out of control.
Fact: Epilepsy is not a one size fits all disorder. Every person experiences seizure activity differently just as everyone who gets a cold experiences them differently.

Myth: Epilepsy is a disease.
Fact: Epilepsy is a disorder, period! The brain produces sudden bursts of electrical energy that disrupt other brain functions and causes a disorder inside the brain.

Myth: An ambulance should be called when someone has a seizure.
Fact: The majority of the time people do not need medical attention. The specific criterion to be followed before calling for help can be found in *Seizure Types and Triggers.* Refer to: *Seizure First Aid*

Myth: All seizures are caused by epilepsy.
Fact: There are many conditions and circumstances that cause seizures. Refer to: *Glossary:* non epileptic seizures, and seizure disorders.

Myth: People who have epilepsy are demon possessed.
Fact: Modern science has *proven* that epilepsy is a neurological disorder. Demon possession is an ancient belief as you are taught by reading *The History of Epilepsy* chapter.

Myth: Brain tumors cause epilepsy.
Fact: Just because a person has a brain tumor does not mean they will have seizures. However tumors may cause epilepsy yet is not a definite end result for someone who has a brain tumor.

Myth: People with epilepsy look different.
Fact: Unless someone with epilepsy is actually having a seizure, there are rare cases that their condition can be determined by features or any other outward signs.

Myth: People with epilepsy aren't allowed to drive.
Fact: Each state has its own laws. Usually, permission to drive legally depends on how much time has passed since the last seizure.

Myth: Women with epilepsy cannot have children.
Fact: Many women can and do have perfectly healthy normal babies.

Myth: Everyone with epilepsy can have control over the seizures. Only people, who don't take their medicine, still have seizures.
Fact: Epilepsy is a chronic medical condition and for some people can be successfully controlled. Some, however, regardless of their efforts continue to be plagued by them. Unfortunately, treatment doesn't work for everyone.

Myth: People with epilepsy can't go to school or college.
Fact: Most people with epilepsy are perfectly capable of attending school and college.

Myth: No one with epilepsy can live a "normal" life.
Fact: Seventy to Eighty percent of all people with epilepsy are seizure free and/or have reasonable control over seizures as a result of proper diagnosis and treatment. Therefore, they live perfectly normal lives.

Myth: People with epilepsy are brain damaged.
Fact: Epilepsy is a disorder of the brain that may or may not be associated with damage to the brain. Brain injuries range from undetectable to disabling. Although brain cells usually do not regenerate, most people can recover substantially. Brain damage, like epilepsy, carries a stigma, and some people may unjustly consider brain-injured patients incompetent.

Myth: Seizures cause brain damage.
Fact: Some people have difficulty with memory and other intellectual functions after a seizure. These problems may be caused by the after

effects of the seizure on the brain, the effects of seizure medication, or both. Usually however, these problems do not mean the brain has been damaged by a seizure.

Myth: Epilepsy is inherited.
Fact: Most cases of epilepsy are not inherited, although some types are passed on through the family. See: *Women and Epilepsy*

Myth: Epilepsy is a barrier to a successful life.
Fact: Epilepsy is perfectly compatible with a healthy, happy, satisfying life. Quality of life may be somewhat affected by the frequency and severity of seizures, side effects from medications, reaction from onlookers to seizures, and other issues that are often associated with or caused by epilepsy.

Myth: Epilepsy is a curse.
Fact: Like asthma, diabetes, and high blood pressure, epilepsy is a medical condition.

Myth: Epilepsy is a lifelong disorder.
Fact: About one quarter of the epilepsy population may develop difficult to control seizures which are likely to require lifelong treatment. However, more than half of childhood forms of epilepsy are outgrown by adulthood. With many forms of epilepsy in children and adults, when the person has been free of seizures for one to three years, medications can often be slowly withdrawn and discontinued under a doctor's supervision.

Myth: Epilepsy surgery is too risky.
Fact: Epilepsy surgery is surely risky. But just like any other operation, there is a small risk of infection or a hemorrhage with the probability of one percent. In general, most patients do extremely well after surgery. See: *Treatment Options*

Myth: People with epilepsy can't fly in planes.
Fact: People with epilepsy can fly just like everyone else! There's absolutely no threat to any type of seizure or epilepsy.

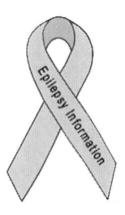

Famous People with Epilepsy

The problem with negativity toward epilepsy could be lessened if we would take the time to tell people about the famous people who had or have epilepsy. Share the names of the famous people in this list with your family and friends. Help them surpass their belief that people with epilepsy are so limited that they don't have the ability to excel or make a difference in life. They will see by the following list, they couldn't be more wrong!

Bud Abbot Comedian (Abbot and Costello)

Neil Abercrombie U.S. Congressman

Alexander the Great General and Macedonian king

Ludwig Van Beethoven Pianist and composer

Buddy Bell Major League baseball player and manager

Hector Berlioz Composer

Napoleon Bonaparte French Emperor

Susan Boyle Scottish singer

Lindsey Buckingham Guitarist and singer in the music group Fleetwood Mac

Lord Byron Anglo-Scottish poet

Julius Caesar Roman Ruler

Lewis Carroll Author of *Alice in Wonderland* and *Through the Looking Glass*. Lewis had temporal lobe epilepsy. The experiences in which Alice encountered, such as when she is falling down a hole, growing or shrinking before her own eyes along with surrounding objects mimicked symptoms of his temporal lobe seizures!

Agatha Christie Author who sold over two billion books!

Jean Clemens Daughter of Mark Twain

Marion Clignet Champion Cyclist

Tony Coelho U.S. Congressman

Ian Curtis Singer and songwriter of the band, *Joy Division*

Dante Author of *The Divine Comedy*

Alan Faneca Football player for Arizona Cardinals

Vincent Van Gogh Artist

Dai Greene Welsh 400 hurdler world champion

George Frederick Handel Composer, pianist

Rick Harrison Reality television star of *Pawn Stars*, Author of *License to Pawn*

Margeaux Hemingway Actress

Gary Howatt Hockey player for New York Islanders

Billy Idol Singer, song writer

Elton John Singer, song writer

Bobby Jones Basketball player

Thom Jones Short stories author of children's books, many included characters with epilepsy

Martin Luther King, Jr. Pastor, Revolutionist

Hal Lanier Baseball player and manager for New York Yankees, San Francisco Giants

Edward Lear English painter, poet

Wally Lewis Australian professional rugby player, team captain

Guy de Maupassant French writer

Deborah McFadden Commissioner, Administrator for Developmental Disabilities

Michelangelo Painter and sculpture artist

Moliere Novelist, writer

Elizabeth Monroe Wife of President James Monroe

Alfred Nobel Swedish inventor of the *Brooklyn Bridge, Lipstick, Love Notes*, and more

Niccolo Paganini Italian violinist

Blaise Pascal French scientist, philosopher, and mathematician

Edgar Allen Poe American poet, short story writer, playwright, editor, literary critic, essayist, and one of the leaders of the *American Romantic Movement*!

Jimmy Reed American blues singer

John Roberts American Chief Justice

Samari Rolle American football player for Baltimore Ravens

Robert Schumann Composer

Sir Walter Scott Literary figure of the romantic period

Kathy Sierra Programming instructor, game developer, co-creator of the *Head First* book series on computer programming

Jonathan Swift Author of *Gulliver's Travels*

Algemon Charles Swinburne English poet

Tchaikovsky Composer

Alfred Lord Tennyson Poet

Leo Tolstoy Russian Novelist, Author of *Anna Karenina,* and *War and Peace*

Harriet Tubman African-American abolitionist

Paul Wade Australian national rugby player, television sports commentator

Greg Walker Baseball player for the Chicago White Sox

Don Craig Wiley Protein-structure biochemist

Kyffin Williams Landscape painter

Neil Young *a.k.a.* **"Shaky"** singer, song writer

The bottom line is famous people with epilepsy have made a significant impact in the world. Epilepsy does not have to limit your potential in life. Everyone has a gift within them. Don't allow epilepsy stop you from expressing your gift. Work hard at doing and being your best.

Personal

Issues

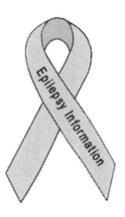

Coping Strategies

Epilepsy can certainly change your life to the point in which you have to "adjust" accordingly. Regardless of the changes, many people live productive and satisfactory lives. It doesn't seem quite as bad if you know what to do and how to do it. It's much easier to live with when you accept it, along with the many unpleasant side effects that come along for the ride.

Denial When you're first diagnosed with epilepsy or lack control over it, it seems the first challenge is accepting the harsh reality. It's not uncommon for the diagnosis to be unacceptable which results in refusing to deal with all the aspects. However, with information and support from your doctor and other epilepsy patients, you can combat some of the frustrating, negative feelings that may be holding you back from your potential. When you accept the fact you have epilepsy, you're empowering yourself. On the other hand, if you deny you have epilepsy you're only causing yourself a great disservice through personal conflict.

When you're in denial, you may lack the desire to take your medications, either correctly or at all. If you deny the treatment your brain desperately needs, you will be taking the chance of inviting more seizure activity not to mention increasing the severity of the seizures.

Denial may also become a reason for you to avoid talking about the many issues you're feeling and dealing with on a regular basis. Therefore, allowing you to suffer from serious depression which can turn into a life threatening situation. Don't allow yourself to fall into the trap of the dark world of depression.

Depression is not the same as the common "feeling down" or the occasional sad times most people experience throughout life. Depression can be a serious threat to your well-being.

Signs of serious depression:
- Consistently fatigued
- Contemplating suicide
- Difficulty sleeping
- Feeling discouraged
- Feeling unloved and rejected
- Inability to concentrate
- Inability to finish a task
- Lack of appetite
- Lack of interest in things you once enjoyed
- Unplanned weight change

If you sense this happening to you, you need to seek help. Talk to your doctor. It's possible your medication may be a part of the problem. Sometimes a medication adjustment will help. "Adjusting" your frame of mind is another way to gain control over depression.

If you suffer from seizures daily which are causing you to barely function, don't give up! There may be treatments you haven't tried. There may even be a treatment in research that's not yet available. It may be the one that will help you gain better control over seizures or better yet, help you become seizure free!

I do understand what it's like to suffer the lack of living a "normal" life. But if you give up, you'll never achieve your dreams. If you ever felt or feel like life with epilepsy is doomed to failure, read the following story:

I was misdiagnosed for three years. I was getting little to no treatment during that time. But thank God I was directed to a reputable epileptologist. She treated me with medications, which included many adjustments and different blends of medications for up to a year. But nothing helped. My epilepsy was out of control which resulted in no less than a dozen seizures daily. The doctors and I decided that surgery was my best option. So I had a right temporal lobectomy and enjoyed seizure free living.

Unfortunately, six months after surgery I started having seizures again. But I was only having two daily! We tried medications to get them under control again with no improvement. So it was obvious a second surgery was the next step. Unfortunately, that surgery didn't cure me either due to the fact a major drainage vein was in the way. However, the seizures were better controlled.

I remained seizure free for several months. When I started having seizures again they were a different type. This time medication was the best treatment! The seizures I was experiencing were few and far between. Due to the surgeries and multiple medication treatments, my life has improved. I'm still taking medication for seizure control. I've had breakthrough seizures which demanded new medications with the typical adjustments. The recent adjustment has been promising.

I hear people's pity statements about how I've been through so much and it's a shame I still have seizures. So I remind them of what it was like way back in the beginning of my battle. It helps them also appreciate how well I'm doing. I want to help people understand that they should be happy for me! I want them to know how much better my life is even with seizure activity. Yes I went through a lot to get to where I am today. But everything I went through was worth it. I've said this dozens of times, "If I had to, I'd do it again, and I did! I have no regrets!"

The lesson you can learn is it takes a positive attitude, patience, and determination. I know it can seem hopeless at times but its only promising to be hopeless *if* you give up. Continue looking toward the future for the right treatment. In other words, always keep your chin up and eyes open!

If you have occasional seizures and some-times feel they're just too hard to deal with, try not to get discouraged. Try to appreciate the fact it's not worse. Yes, seizures are emotionally draining and can be physically painful. You have every right to be upset. But if you're able to do the things you desire most of the time, try to be thankful. If you feel your life isn't productive enough, think about your situation differently. Let me help you . . .

Do you go to school or work and get out amongst your friends? Do you get through days maybe even weeks without a seizure? If your answers are yes, you have something to be grateful for. You certainly have the right to want a better life. But instead of looking at life in a hopeless manner adjust your frame of mind. Find a way to be thankful. If you struggle doing so, let me help you again . . .

Can you walk, talk, read, think independently, and eat a delicious meal? Then you have a reason to be thankful. Think about the precious little babies that started their life with epilepsy. Beautiful babies that grew into innocent children who never sat up on their own, spoke a word, walked, nor savored the many delicious foods everyone else enjoys due to the fact they have to get their nutrition through a feeding tube. They never experienced life as you know it. When you look at it that way you can surely recognize you have a reason to be grateful. See: *Children's Epilepsy*. Both the information and stories are awe inspiring. You'll be able to see and appreciate life differently. Maybe in a way you never had before.

Try to enjoy each day you sit up, walk, eat a large nutritious flavorful meal, and talk your heart out to others. Look away from the times that are emotionally draining and concentrate on the positive times in your life. After all, it could be worse *and* it will get better once you alter your frame of mind.

Now that you feel better about yourself, get involved with other people who have epilepsy. Help them see themselves and their situation in a better light. Suggest that they visit online epilepsy social sites, contact the Epilepsy Foundation, and/or join or start a local support group.

Reach out your hand and help someone else who is struggling. When you help others, there's a beautiful feeling that stirs up inside you. It not only gives you a reason to thrive but is an excitable joyous reason to look forward to every day. But don't take my word for it, try it and see for yourself! See: *Epilepsy Friends*

Another way to gain control over despair is to stay productive. Not only is keeping busy, good for combating hopelessness but it'll also be good for stimulating your brain in a healthy way. Go for walks with a friend, read a book, study subjects that intrigue you, and . . .

Dance as if no one were looking!

Sing as if no one were listening!

Live as if it were you last day!

(Irish Proverb)

Now you know what to do. It's up to you to get started!

Self worth Look around at your peers. Are they acting like they are fortunate to have healthy bodies? Do they complain a lot about their features? Do they appreciate every seizure free day in which they have the luxury to enjoy? Of course they don't think about how precious every day is without a seizure but you do! You value life in a way they can't possibly imagine. In a very unique way, you have more than them. You know how to appreciate life especially every seizure free day. They can't appreciate that sort of enjoyment! So the bottom line is it's up to you to make the best of your life. Enjoy those special moments that are rare and precious.

If you struggle with your self-worth, step back and, see yourself in a different light. The following is an analogy to help you see the "big picture." See yourself as a newly released movie with great reviews. Everyone wants to see it. They expect to love it wholeheartedly. The beginning of the movie is bright and exciting. It's loved by the entire audience. Then the dark scary scene comes, one that's disliked by most. But after that scene is over, the movie is exciting again and the people are enjoying it. As a matter of fact, most of them walk away saying it was the best movie they ever saw! They want to go back and see it again! They didn't care there was an unpleasant scary scene. The movie as a whole was still enjoyed, loved, and desired.

Picture yourself as that movie. The seizure is the dark scene in which the viewers feared and disliked. But when it's all over, you're still loved and desired. You're the movie that everyone runs telling their friends about how great you are! Take time to sit back and see yourself that way. The seizures you have are just the dark scenes of your life. You're still the person who everyone wants to see. They know that even the dark scary scene is just a small portion of the entire you. It's time you recognize that, too!

Punishment is not the cause of epilepsy. Do you feel epilepsy is a form of punishment? Punishment is a *type of disciplinary action for a wrong doing*. You have not been personally chosen to suffer for any wrong doing. You have not done anything wrong to deserve or earn epilepsy. You're living in a world that promises hardship no matter how good, or bad you are, or by your status in life.

Do you catch yourself asking the ever so popular question, "Why me?" Instead of asking why me, ask, "What for?" When you ask "Why me?" you can get distracted and only see the negative side. You can end up wallowing in self pity. But when you ask the question, "What for?" you'll slowly get an answer because there's a purpose for every adversity in life. Ask yourself, "What can I learn from this situation? How can I take my affliction and turn it into something good?" You are certainly experiencing a hardship that is more than challenging. However, challenges can be an asset to improve who you are and turn you into a better stronger person. Yes, it's far from pleasant, but if you become a better person due to it, you'll no longer see yourself as being punished.

So even though epilepsy can drag you down physically and emo-tionally, you have the power to turn it into something good. No, I don't like what I'm going through either but I do like the way it changed me. I'm a better person. We're not being punished, we're being improved! We need to thrive on that rather than keep asking the unanswerable question, "Why me?"

Seizure free setbacks can be one of the hardest issues to cope with. When you're enjoying a seizure free life and everything's going great, a setback can cause a serious "melt down." You might feel like you fell into a dark hole. But when you have breakthrough seizures, it doesn't mean you're back to square one. The first thing you need to do is contact your doctor. You might just need a medication adjustment with your present medication and/or add another medication to your present regimen. With time, and a few adjustments, you may become seizure free again.

Shame is an emotion you may be experiencing. Shame means, *strong sense of guilt, embarrassment, unworthiness* or *disgrace*. None of the words which define the word shame applies to anyone with epilepsy, including you! Since the words in the definition take on a lot of meaning of their own, they're defined also.

> **Embarrassment:** *To cause to feel self-conscious or ill at ease.* Did you catch the key word, "cause?" Are <u>you</u> *causing* yourself to be ill at ease or has the outside world inflicted it on you? There's absolutely no reason to feel embarrassed. I know it is uncomfortable thinking about the possibility of having a seizure in front of people not to mention strangers. But you have no reason to be embarrassed if you do. You have a health condition.

> I met a woman who came to my church for the first time completely bald due to chemotherapy treatments. She bravely and unashamedly subjected herself to a host of strangers yet never appeared uncomfortable. She did not show any signs of embarrassment. She held her head high. She impressed me in a way that I realized if she could do it so could I! And if I can do it, so can you!

> **Disgrace:** *Loss of honor, respect or reputation.* You don't lose honor from a battle with epilepsy any more than an injured soldier

does from battle wounds. Respect and reputation have nothing to do with health issues. They are defined by personality, honesty, consideration, and faithfulness, etc. So don't allow feelings of disgrace get intertwined with your health issues, whether it's epilepsy or anything else. Hold your head up and be proud of who you are.

Guilt: *Being responsible for an offensive wrongdoing, guilty behavior, responsible for or chargeable for a blameworthy act, at fault.* You cannot avoid a seizure just because it would upset or negatively affect someone. Having a seizure is not your fault or a moral wrong! When you're guilty of something you did intentionally, you should feel guilty. But that's obviously not the case here, so what wrong do you need to admit? You haven't committed a crime! Can you imagine standing in front of a judge saying, "Yes Sir, I am in the wrong because I had a seizure in front of that person? I'm guilty as charged!" When you look at it that way, doesn't it seem silly! After all, *you are innocent!*

If you don't necessarily feel guilty, just sad because you think you may have upset someone during a seizure, you don't need to apologize. For example, you are somewhere with dozens of people such as school, work or a meeting and the teacher/speaker is in the middle of their session. Then you suddenly have a seizure. When you "come to," you notice a lot of people around you.

My guess is you'll do what I've done too many times to count and say, "I'm so sorry." But if you get the same response as I usually did, you'll realize it's definitely unnecessary to apologize. People will probably respond by saying something like, "It's okay. You didn't do anything wrong. Are you okay? Can I get you a drink of water or something?" They won't understand why you're apologizing because they know you didn't have any control over the seizure.

The bottom line is you do not have to apologize!

Unworthy: *Insufficient in worth, undeserving.* You're just as worthy as everyone else in this world! Having epilepsy does not change your worth, period! If everyone in this world expressed guilt, embarrassment, un-worthiness, and disgrace due to a health condition where would this world be? You cannot afford to allow such emotions control you. You need to take that negative energy, and turn it around so it can positively improve your world. You need to see yourself as special. Don't see yourself as odd, see yourself as unique.

Driving privileges When you have your driving privileges taken away from you or are restricted from ever getting them, it's no big secret it can be extremely difficult to deal with. Yes, it's definitely hard to depend on others and at times causes a dilemma. It's indeed hard to work and run errands. However, states must consider both the public's and patient's safety.

While you're waiting for chance to get behind the wheel again or even for the first time, remember driving is a privilege not a right! Be thankful you don't have to walk a tight wire! After all, would you take the risk of driving to obtain your personal freedom if it wasn't against the law? Would you struggle one way or the other? Try to be thankful the government has helped you balance the risks with personal freedom.

Depending on your state's laws, you may be permitted to drive legally. But just because you're legally permitted to drive, doesn't mean you should drive everywhere you want *just because*. You need to be honest with yourself. You know it can be a game of "Russian roulette" each time you get behind the wheel. There's no guarantee a seizure won't breakthrough. Be sure the trip to the store is necessary not just because you feel like getting out. Look at your vehicle as a means of transportation only, not as a way to get from here to there *just because*. In other words, be responsible with your driving privileges. If it's legal for you to drive, it's up to you to balance your need for independence and safety.

Keep this in mind. Removing driving privileges is not solely for people with epilepsy. There are many other medical conditions which remove a person's driving privileges at their doctor's discretion. They include heart conditions, dementia, Alzheimer's disease, diabetes, stroke, arthritis, eye problems (cataract's and glaucoma), hearing disorders, Parkinson's disease, and other neurological disorders. So there you have it! All the conditions mentioned are a danger to the person behind the wheel as well as other drivers and pedestrians. You can maintain your dignity if you look at the situation in the right perspective. It's all about safety.

A lobbying effort by patients and doctors has produced a step-by-step reduction in the period needed to be seizure free which has allowed for more exceptions for driving. Therefore, the laws are growing more liberalized. Seizure free periods in the U.S. ranges from three months to two years and many states leave it discretionary. Some states might require intermittent medical evaluation. Since the laws are different from one state to the next, it's up to you to do your homework. Start by checking with your doctor. If you are restricted from driving, every state offers the privilege of a photo identification card.

If it's legal for you to drive, consider making the following personal commitments before driving:
- Take your medication *on time.*
- Do not to drive when *excessively tired.*
- Don't drive when you've been *exposed to a "trigger."*
- Be honest with your doctor and report all seizure activity since your previous appointment.
- Don't drive somewhere just "because."
- Don't be too proud to ask someone to drive you somewhere when you're already out with your car and feel "unsteady." What's worse? A little humility or an accident that can harm, maim or kill you along with someone else who is innocently on the same road at the same time.

Income issues Finding a way to survive monetarily can be a dilemma, whether you're looking for your first job or replacing the income from the job you once had. But no matter what your dilemma is, there are ways to resolve the issues.

Employment: Many people with epilepsy do hold jobs successfully especially those with excellent seizure control. If you have occasional, or fairly frequent seizures, that might make your job hunt a little more difficult but not impossible. Unfortunately, there is still a stigma attached to epilepsy which may cause discrimination. But fear not, the government has taken a stand to protect people with "disabilities." The *Americans with Disabilities Act*, which is a wide-ranged federal civil rights law that prohibits discrimination against people with disabilities in the workplace.

Choosing your line of work is not as hard as you might expect. If you are not permitted to drive, you should obviously not get a job with dangerous machinery. There are a few jobs that are not open to people with epilepsy, because they are particularly dangerous. When you're considering a career, think about how well the seizures are controlled, the type and frequency, and the impact they might have on any particular job.

If your seizure control is almost completely reliable, then basically all jobs are an open opportunity. Before you start searching for your job, take time to decide what type of *long-term* employment you desire. You may be eligible for government-run employment programs that provide job counseling, training, placement, and transportation allowance.

Disability benefits: If seizure activity affects your ability to work you should file for disability benefits. Do not hire an attorney right away! You may win your case without one. If you are turned down, file an appeal immediately, and hire an attorney who *specializes in disability cases*, and is *paid on contingency* (paid only if you win your case). It's customary to pay the lawyer a percentage of your claim payment.

Take note, if you're awarded the benefits after an appeal you will receive your income benefits from the *initial filing date*. Therefore, if you lose the first time, don't start the process over. Simply file an appeal and continue the process! If you are deemed eligible for disability benefits and have dependent children under the age of 18, they are also eligible. Be sure to notify your case worker so you will receive payment for your children as well.

Marriage There is absolutely no reason why you can't get married. The choice of marriage is personal. People with epilepsy have the same right to get married as everyone else in the world! There's nothing to stop you from enjoying one of the greatest pleasures in life.

Epilepsy should not interfere with your marriage. Even though epilepsy can be a negative aspect in your life, it can also be a blessing in a marriage with a strong foundation! If you allow it to make you, your spouse, and your relationship stronger, you'll live a happy long life together and enjoy the "hidden" blessings. I know this from personal experience. My marriage has improved incredibly since epilepsy entered our lives. Now, a decade later, we are happier and more convinced that we belong together. I know without a doubt, I'm married to my soul mate because he lovingly, willingly, and patiently accepted my epilepsy. I couldn't ask for more. You shouldn't expect less.

Anyone who says you shouldn't marry because you have epilepsy is a fool! That's as foolish as saying you shouldn't get married because you have diabetes! Some people will try to convince you, that you shouldn't or won't be able to have children. Anyone that thinks that needs to get educated because they don't have a clue what they're talking about! Don't trust the average person's comments to alter any life changing decisions. Talk to your epileptologist, the Epilepsy Foundation, and/or friends who also have epilepsy.

Sexual Activity: Your sexual activity doesn't need to disappear because you have epilepsy. Most people have a healthy satisfying sex life. Even with poorly controlled epilepsy, there is a *rare* chance that a seizure would be caused by sexual activity. Some males report impotence and lack of desire. Some females report painful inter-course which may be due to dryness therefore, lubricants may be able to help.

Many problems involving sex are *psychosocial* by nature. Acute or chronic stress, low self-esteem, and the fear of seizing during sex can interrupt the natural flow of sexual activity. However, some AEDs have been proven to be the cause since they can sometime affect areas of the brain which is responsible for sexuality. They are also known to cause changes in hormone metabolism. If you're experiencing any problems, don't hesitate to discuss it with your doctor. Many times the problem can be easily alleviated.

Stress Relievers

Even if you have come to terms with epilepsy, it doesn't mean it won't add stress to your life. Since stress is synonymous with epilepsy, there needs to be a few avenues to help gain control over all the havoc it can cause in your life.

Cry. Crying releases a great deal of emotional stress. Keep in mind males have the need and right to cry, too! Don't fall for the American belief that if you're a male and cry, you're a sissy. Actually, it's quite the opposite. If you cry when it's not acceptable, that proves you're strong because you're willing to go against the flow! Go for it!

Get involved in sports or similar activities. One very effective way to work out stress is to move your body. It's not a big secret that getting active is good for combating stress. Playing a sport does not have to be aggressive. Even if you're restricted from physical activities, it doesn't mean you can't engage in an activity that will distract you and physically relieve you. Taking a walk with a friend can give you the opportunity to exercise and verbally vent at the same time.

Read. Reading a magazine, book, or internet sites will "take you away" from the world in which you are trying to escape from.

Enjoy a pet. Research has shown that heart attack victims who have pets live longer. Even watching fish swim around in a tank can relax away your stress! House pets have always been known to be soothing to the nerves. After all, dogs are called man's best friend for a reason! Just about all house pets enjoy snuggling and petting which have been proven to reduce high blood pressure and reduce stress.

Listen to soft music. Music can be a powerful tool because it increases production of serotonin in the brain. Serotonin is a chemical in the brain known for its calming affects. Playing music in the background, even though you are busy during some other activity and are not aware of the music, still calms your nerves which in turn reduces stress levels.

Use aromatherapy. Aromatherapy has been around for thousands of years and has supplied welcomed relief to millions of people. It has evolved little over the years and is one of the purest forms of relaxation in which Cleopatra enjoyed! Simply light aromatic candles, use aromatic plug-ins, and/or enjoy smokeless wax warmers. If you're a guy, don't be too critical about trying aromatherapy. There are many scents that aren't "girly." For instance, you can enjoy the scent of apple pie or mixed berries. There are many "around the house" scents available. Find the perfect scent, and enjoy the stress relief!

Turn down the lights! Bright lights are demanding. When you turn down the lights, a calm feeling overflows your mind and body.

Watch television. There are plenty of game shows to cause you to think hard which will distract you from your pressures. A good movie or comedy series are also good ideas. Avoid watching the news. There's always more bad than good!

Make a craft or any DIY project. You can distract yourself from your struggles by involving yourself in a project that takes a lot of thought. You can make something for yourself or as a gift. Research online, to find the many projects that will work best for you. The beauty with the internet is there's a world of options that never run out!

Write letters, cards, poems, etc. Writing works for several reasons. It's a great form of distraction, and an outlet to express emotions. Most importantly, it takes you away from the "world" in which you're trying to escape. Sending thank you cards to people who have supported and helped you is a great outlet. It makes you feel good as you return the good given to you. People feel special when they receive something that's been thought through and written with pen and paper! It's a personal compliment to physically write a card or letter and is so much more appreciated than you can imagine.

Laugh! Laughing is a great avenue for stress relief. It decreases levels of stress hormones like adrenal and cortisol which causes endorphin levels to rise. Humor also has psychological benefits. It makes it easier to take things lightly, breaking away from stress producing thoughts, increasing your sense of satisfaction, and making your life feel more meaningful. It also helps you in relating to others around you. If you aren't able to go out much, watch a good comedy movie, series, and/or go online and read comedy websites.

Physical affection works wonders! Studies have shown physical touch is a great stress reliever. Everyone needs affection. Easy ways of filling that need is merely by getting a hug, gentle kiss, or even a simple hand shake. So get as much loving as you can from your family and friends! If your loved ones have alienated you due to seizure activity, you can still receive the affection you need. The best place to get affection is a place where it's needed just as bad. Try a nursing home. People in nursing homes are often affectionately neglected and desperately in need of physical touch. It's highly unlikely that you'll be turned away. The affection you share will not only help you but the patients as well.

Vent:
- Talk to friends.
- Contact the Epilepsy Foundation.
- Call a family member!
- Make a phone call or "house call!"
- Go to online epilepsy social sites.
- Discuss your concerns with your doctor. You may be experiencing stress over something which can be remedied.

"Seizure proof" your home. Since you're subject to injury due to seizures, it's important to protect yourself so you can enjoy the comforts of your home. Worrying about getting hurt can certainly cause stress.

Living Space:

- Lay carpet with a heavy pile and padding throughout the house, including staircases. If you rent your home, add area carpets for extra padding.
- Place pads on any furniture that has sharp corners or are potentially dangerous.
- Use chairs that have padded arms.
- Use electric and home appliance devices that have automatic shut-off switches.
- When you buy furniture, choose pieces that have rounded corners, preferably padded.
- If you use a space heater, choose one that won't tip over or turns off if it is tipped over. Also try to get one with a grate that doesn't get hot.

Bathroom:

- For extreme cases, install a bathtub seat with a safety strap so you won't fall down.
- Make sure the bathroom doors open outward rather than inward so they can be opened by someone else if you need assistance.
- Take showers only. No baths!
- Turn down the water heater to prevent scalding.

Kitchen:

- If you use a stove, use the back burners only.
- Slide hot food containers along the counter.
- Use a cart to move hot food from one room to the next rather than pick them up.
- When possible, use a microwave oven rather than a stove.

Take a vacation! You don't have to work to need a vacation. Staying in your normal everyday world can be stressful. Everyone needs to take a vacation once in a while! We all need a "change of scene" But keep in mind, when you have epilepsy, it's very important to plan ahead! If you want to be able to relax, you need to make sure you've done everything necessary in the event of a seizure so you can truly relax.

Get the name, telephone number, and exact directions:

- Hospital(s)
- Pharmacy
- Ambulance stations (If you have extreme difficulty with seizure activity, it would be wise to talk to the paramedics at the beginning of your vacation).

Carry the following information with you at all times:

- List of allergies
- Name and telephone number for:
  - ► Neurologist/epileptologist
  - ► Family doctor
  - ► Emergency contact (at least two)
- Your medication schedule. Write each medication, the time of day it's taken, and the dosage amount each time. For example:

1. medication #1 (200 mg. a.m., 200 mg. p.m., and 400 mg. bed time)
2. medication #2 (100 mg. a.m., 100 mg. p.m., 200 mg. bed)

Be sure to:

- Wear a medical alert bracelet that has a "compartment" to hold vital information. (I strongly encourage you to purchase one, whether you go on vacation, or not).
- Keep your rescue medication with you at all times. (Take a plentiful amount).
- Take a seven day pill box organizer with daily detachable compartments. There are two very good reasons for this:
1. You can take a daily box with you if you go out for the day.
2. You will be able to check if you took your medications.

- Take *written* prescriptions. (For the unlikely chance you'd lose your medications or run out).
- Enjoy your vacation!

Faith/Prayer As humans, we can be too proud and favor taking on our problems alone. We have a tendency to think if we seek help that means we're weak! That couldn't be farthest from the truth! After all, you're seeking help from a doctor and feel completely comfortable doing so! When you rely on God, you'll be able to deal with all the issues that are dragging you down. *Come to Me, you who are weary and heavy burdened, and I will give you rest.* Matthew 11:28. It doesn't say, He'll take away all your burdens, it says, He will be there for you and help you rest.

As you grow in faith, the battles which appear to be as big as Goliath will no longer feel gigantic, unmovable, and overwhelming. As you take every burden to God in prayer, the heaviness of epilepsy will feel less empowering. Your prayers may not take away your problems, however they will be easier to handle because you're giving them to God. The beauty of prayer is that God is always ready and willing to listen anytime of the day or night. He doesn't look at you with condemning eyes because you have epilepsy. You're His child in whom He loves dearly. Don't take His love for granted.

Communicate with Him about everything. Follow His lead through Christ who prayed every day, when He was creeping up on His moment of death on the cross. He didn't run away crying. He went with His disciples to the garden of Gethsemane and said to them, "Sit here while I go over there to pray." That was just hours prior to His crucifixion in which He was completely aware. If He was able to stop and pray shortly before His arrest and demise, you can surely do the same with your situation.

Trust in the Lord with all your heart and lean not on your own understanding. In all your ways acknowledge Him, and He shall direct your path. Proverbs 3:5 – 6

True Stories

I have a daughter with epilepsy. As a parent of a child with epilepsy, I cope in many ways. First and foremost is with God's help. I believe for me, it is God that gives me the strength to cope. I also try to stay optimistic and hopeful, focusing on the positive not the negative. But most of all from support of family and friends. Surrounding yourself with caring and supportive people is very comforting. Knowing you're not alone!
Wanda, Myrtle Beach SC

I am 27 years old and was diagnosed with epilepsy at the age of 19. I am able to go through life with epilepsy due to the support I get from family, friends, and my beloved fiancé. During my available time, I play speed ball, a fast paced version of paint ball in which teamwork results in winning. If I did not have anyone or anything to support my epilepsy, I don't know how my life would be.
F. Hernandez, White Plains NY

Coping is hard some days, but I have fallen into a routine. I have family and friends who I know I can count on for rides. My job is easy to deal with. The hardest part is getting back and forth for all my trainings and supervisions. I went to school for carpentry but it's virtually useless. Who knows what I'd do without the job I have now. It relies mainly on the least reliable part of my body, my brain! But I just keep poking along doing what I have to, to get by. I truly hope the surgery works out for me, so my wife and daughter don't have to cope anymore.
B. Webster, ME

Pretty simply, I cope day by day. It is a challenge some days, especially the days when I feel discouraged. I have my good days and my bad days. But I take the support I get from family and friends very dearly. To cope with epilepsy cannot be to pretend it isn't there. We don't have that option. In my daily life, I take my medications, try to get enough sleep, eat enough, and try to keep my stress level down. And I try to remember to not take it so seriously. I feel like I have to have a sense of humor about it. If I can't control it, at least I can control how I react to it.

K. Eastin, Waite Park MN

I cope by believing in God. As far as the environment that surrounds my epilepsy, I overlook people's ignorance! I try to make the best of the situation by looking at everything in a positive way. When I couldn't drive, I thought, well at least I don't have to pay insurance, taxes or worry about getting speeding tickets!

T. Lambert, Georgetown SC

Coping with epilepsy is sometimes harder on some days than others but so are a lot of other things in life. The main thing I keep in mind is epilepsy is a part of my life however it does not define who I am. Everyone is unique in some way or another. People with asthma have asthma attacks, people with diabetes have to monitor their sugar. I have seizures but life does go on. The worst thing you can do is let seizures keep you from leading a normal life because you will just feel worse in the end.

I make it a habit to do something once a week to relax. Exercise, meditation, or a nice massage is a couple of ways to relax. I forget about the seizures! The most important way to cope is to have a strong support system and an even stronger faith. My family, friends, and doctors serve as my support system when I have a problem. More importantly my faith helps me cope when I am feeling my worst. I

have learned to reassure myself when I feel scared because life is too short. I do what I can, to control the seizures, and leave the rest up to God.
A. Jewell, Santa Fe TX

As a parent of nine year old, with epilepsy, I have gone through many methods of coping. I started with burying my head in a pillow and crying. Then I realized that was not helping me or Bailey. I use researching and talking to cope now. By researching and using the internet. I have been able to come to terms and realize we are not alone. I can also find information that helps me when I speak to the doctor. It helps not just me but Bailey, also because I can give him solutions and reasons for certain things that we may not have known in the past.

I have coped with the bad days by talking, talking, talking!People probably get tired of listening to me but it makes me feel better! I do not hide anything. I share everything in regards to Bailey, and what he is going through. It gives me a great sense of security for me to know that others around him know what is going on because I feel people will be more understanding. If people around him under-stand what is going on, I can deal with everything else. The only thing I cannot deal with and cannot cope with is, when other people blame bad behavior or a behavior disorder for some of the problems he has. The way I have learned to cope is talk, talk, talk!
T. Anasenes, Elgin IL

I was raised going to church and *having faith in God*. When I had my first seizure in ninth grade in front of my peers, it took the life out of me. I got bitter because I couldn't figure out why God would do this to me. *But after I got over that pitiful attitude and gave it to Him, I realized He didn't cause it, He allowed it for my good.* Some people think I'm crazy when I tell them that, but it's not a guessing game, it's a fact. I am a better, stronger person because of my epilepsy. I'm a more focused and determined person. I don't take life for granted. It feels good to have the balance of my friends who respect me because of my mindset and faith rather than disrespect from my peers who fear me.

Carol Anne, Chattanooga TN

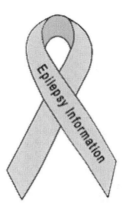

Memory Issues and Solutions

Can you remember when you had a memory?! Memory issues are one of the most talked about symptoms of epilepsy, and rightfully so! The memory process is much more than short term and long term. Your brain is far from simplistic. It is a complicated precious organ which helps to define you, and provides you with one of your most precious senses, your memory.

Do you catch yourself asking questions like . . .
- Why can't I remember how to spell a simple everyday word?
- Why can I remember what I did when I was a little kid but I can't remember a telephone conversation from yesterday?
- Why can't I remember people's names when I've known them for a long time?
- Why does my mind go blank when I'm trying to express a thought that I'm completely prepared to say?
- Why can't I remember something even though I studied it for hours?

The answer is because you're like the rest of us who have epilepsy. Memory loss is a part of our condition but it doesn't have to become a major factor in our lives. Just because it's a major challenge doesn't mean we can't overcome it and be productive. If you exercise some of the following techniques, you'll be able to handle the memory struggle head on.

You are not alone, if you:
- Forget what you've just been told
- Forget people's names
- Forget where you placed something
- Get lost in familiar places
- Forget a change in routine
- Forget to do something important
- Simply forget just about anything

If you wonder what *causes* memory loss, you're not alone. Doctors aren't 100% sure but it's believed, seizures and/or medication are the main culprits.

There are many problems which will stem from your lack of memory because it doesn't only affect you but everyone in your life as well. Should you feel guilty? Absolutely not! You should do quite the opposite. Accept the fact that a poor memory is a part of epilepsy and your life. Since it not only affects you but also the people in your life, try to help them understand and accept it as well.

Just as it's frustrating for you, it can be frustrating for them, also. So as you expect them to accept and understand this major shortcoming in your life, be equally patient with them when they have moments of frustration. The best way to understand the way they feel is to mentally put yourself in their "shoes." Try to imagine how you'd feel if the "shoe was on the other foot." Then work together, and attempt to make this issue less painful and irritating.

However, if you're loved ones are more than frustrated and tend to treat you disrespectfully, stand your ground! Let them know you deserve respect despite your adversity. Don't settle for mistreatment due to your memory loss. You can't help it, so it's important to urge them to understand you can't change it. It's a major characteristic of epilepsy. Expect and insist on respect, after you've given them an appropriate amount of time to adjust. Then stick up for yourself!

Remind your loved ones if they love you they need to love all of you. Accent on the fact, they need to love each and every part of you, shortcomings and all!

MEMORY TECHNIQUES

There are many ways to help you remember valuable information. Some are helped by physical aids and others depend on stretching your memory capacity. Either way, remembering is possible. You just have to know the "tricks." Search for the techniques that work best for you, and enjoy remembering the bits and pieces of your life!

PHYSICAL AIDS

- If you read your email faithfully, email yourself! If it's short, simply write the message in the subject line.
- Send yourself a voice mail.
- Utilize any electronic device you have!
- Keep a journal or diary.
- Make a scrapbook for special events.
- Write things down on a memo board.
- Keep a notepad in your pocket, purse, or glove compartment.
- Use bright colored highlighters to color code important dates on a wall calendar. For example: use orange for doctor appointments, green for "to do" dates, etc. Another benefit to color coding is you'll be able to quickly scan your important dates by color rather than having to read everything!
- Keep track of your appointments and personal notes in a daily planner.
- Keep important information saved in your electronic devices *and* on paper! The best way to make sure you don't lose your important information is to *save it both digitally and physically*.
- Don't write important details on pieces of paper and throw them on the kitchen table, counter, or anywhere else! Keep them all in one place or you'll likely lose them.
- Keep a notepad and pen at your bedside.

- Keep a journal to document and keep track of details regarding information, especially over the phone, which are unique for a specific situation. You may need to refer back to them in the future and won't be able to remember the details or even the situation itself.
- Keep a personal journal of your life. Adults think it's sweet or cute for a little girl to write in her diary. Yet it proves to be precious when she's older as the "little" things bring a smile on her face, a giggle to her heart, and a moment she'll treasure forever. You can enjoy that same feeling if you write about the "small" events that take place in your life. It may come as a surprise how fun or precious they'll prove to be when someday you reflect back on them.
- *For short term, such as for the next day, place reminder notes around the house:*
  - With your medication
  - On your bathroom mirror
  - On the kitchen counter and table
  - On your dresser
  - With your shoes
  - On your microwave
  - At your computer
  - On your refrigerator
  - With your keys
  - On or next to your phone
  - With your wallet or pocket book
  - On the door in which you use to exit your home
  - On your car seat
  - Anywhere you see every day

Try not to depend on physical aids all the time. There's nothing wrong with using physical aids but using them only may be somewhat disabling to your memory.

Methods to Remember to Take Your Medication:

- Keep your medication in a pill box organizer with individual daily boxes that have four compartments (it'll be easy to take your medication with you and check if you took each dose).
- Wear an alarm watch.
- Use your cell phone alarm.
- When at home, use an alarm clock, timer on your microwave and stove.

Keep your rescue medication in your pocket or purse in case you take your medication too late or miss a dose.

Stay put!

Always keep the same items in the same place! You'll know where to find them every time. That's almost a guarantee! If you move them, you'll lose them or outright frustrate yourself wishing you didn't move them! Avoid the irritation of hunting for things. Give them a home and always put them back where they belong!

Bundle!

You undoubtedly hear about "bundling" in commercials but did you ever consider it as a memory tactic? Bundling can be used for preparation to ensure you don't forget a single thing! For instance, if you have to be ready for an activity which includes a lot of items, just bundle them together, literally!

For example, if you're leaving early in the morning for school, work, or any other activity in which you'll be gone the entire day, it's in your best interest to prepare the evening before. You need to be ready to get dressed, put on your deodorant, brush your teeth, wash your face, (ladies put on your makeup, and fix your hair), eat, and anything else that's a typical activity of your morning routine. But if you have to move fast, you can easily forget something, like brush your teeth or put on your deodorant! Since that's an unpleasant thought, you're better off to bundle everything together.

All you have to do to organize the day is gather everything together the night before. Have your toothbrush, deodorant, hair products, makeup, wash cloth, and whatever else you need all in one place. Let's face it, when you're in a hurry you have a greater chance of forgetting something. If you need or want to take other things, either put them with all your other items or put them together in a tote bag, a pocket book, brief case, or whatever item you choose at the door in which you'll be exiting.

Bundle your medication, breakfast, and anything else that helps you get the day started. Put your medication next to your coffee maker and mug, have the coffee maker filled and ready to turn on and brew. If you prefer tea, put the tea bag in the mug! For either coffee or tea, have your spoon, sugar, and creamer (if powdered) right next to the coffee maker, stove or microwave. If you prefer liquid creamer or milk with your hot drink, that's a perfect place to put your bundled breakfast. Put your creamer, breakfast items, lunch, bottled water (to take your medicine during the day), and any other refrigerated food all together *on the first shelf*, ready to grab and eat.

For example: if you want a bagel with butter and cream cheese, and an orange put them with the creamer so everything's in one spot. Have the orange peeled and sectioned ahead of time. Just in case you run late, have a couple of breakfast bars in your bag. As for your lunch and bottled water it's right there with everything else, so as soon as you lay eyes on them, put them in or with the package you plan to take along. The idea is to be ready to do everything in a snap. You should be ready to grab and go without trying to organize and remember a single thing. During the moment, whether in the morning, afternoon or evening, it can be memory free, stress free, and easy simply by bundling. Trust me it works beautifully!

MENTAL AIDS

There are many mental ways to memorize information. The following suggestions are just a few of the many options. You may have already tried some of the following. Maybe you even created some of your own!

Focus

Stop what you're doing, and pay attention! You may think you forgot what you've been told. But instead, you were "hearing" rather than "listening" to what was said. You may have given a head nod and possibly an automatic reply such as "okay." Hearing and listening are different! Anyone can hear but when you listen, you specifically pay attention! When someone's talking to you, stop what you're doing and listen. *Specifically reply to them*. Repeat back what you're expected to remember. Concentrate and tune in to what you heard.

If you have to find your way through a big building with corridors which look alike, *focus* on the signs, pictures on the walls, aisle numbers, elevators, and of course, the left and right turns, if applicable.

When you're in a big store, especially one your unfamiliar with, study the physical items on the shelves and item sections such as technology, office products, etc.

Become a "Backseat" Driver

If you don't drive, and catch yourself thinking or saying, "I can't remember how to get there," even though it's not a completely uncommon route, it may be because you're not paying attention.

My friend's house is just a half hour away. It's not in a big city where there are a lot of roads. It takes about four roads to get there but I never pay attention so I wouldn't know how to get there if I had to! I wouldn't even recognize her house if I passed it! I recently decided, I'm going to focus on the *road signs* and *land marks* to learn the way. Then I'm going to become a "backseat driver" and give the driver directions on how to get there! I decided to practice this tactic regularly. I believe it'll work so I'm passing it on to you!

Meditate

In order to move your short term memory into long term, you need to pay very close attention to *your thoughts*. Hide away in a quiet room where you can remove all outside interference such as television, telephone, and other diversions. Take control over your mind. Think specifically about what you want to remember. Intentionally concentrate on one subject. Don't allow your mind to wander.

Repetition

Listen Use electronic devices. If it's practical, get other people to repeat it you.

Verbalize Whatever you're trying to remember, say it out loud even if it means talking to *yourself!*

Visualize If you want to remember something physical, keep viewing it directly or picturing it in your "mind's eye." People in general tend to remember things they can see.

Read The more often you read something the easier it is to remember. Don't hesitate to read it out loud. That will keep you from "drifting" away into other thoughts. It's also "bundling!" You'll be focusing, listening, verbalizing, and visualizing simply by reading the words you see! So if reading's possible, it's the best technique because you'll be using four techniques at one time!

Music, Rhythm, and Jingles

Just like you learned the alphabet, childhood poems such as "Twinkle, Twinkle, Little Star," and commercial "jingles" like "Rice – A – Roni, the San Francisco Treat" or "I am stuck on Band-Aid cause Band-Aid's stuck on me!" You can learn to remember your own words by simply using the same method. As soon as you hear the music and rhythm, you will easily remember the words that go along with them. The beauty is, all you need to do to make your own jingle is insert the words you want to remember!

Develop Consistency

If you want to make sure you'll never miss a step, do the same thing in the same way every time! In other words, make it a habit to become consistent with certain activities and *never* change the order. For instance, always go from left to right, top to bottom, first to last, front to back, Sunday through Saturday, small to big or whatever is appropriate for the task and stay with the sequence every time.

Abbreviations and Acronyms

It's not a big secret that acronyms, abbreviations, including numbers, and symbols work especially well together. After all, we hear and see them often enough that we recognize them as if they were words. We use them in texting, email, and everyday conversations.

Abbreviations

Work great with, letters, numbers, and symbols because they make it shorter, practical, and at times more fun. The more fun you make them, the easier they'll be to remember. You most likely know the following:

- l.o.l. **l**augh **o**ut **l**oud
- a.s.a.p. **a**s **s**oon **a**s **p**ossible
- b.f.n. **b**ye **f**or **n**ow
- b.r.b. **b**e **r**ight **b**ack
- ?4u **q**uestion **f**or **y**ou
- gr8 **gr**eat
- ttyl **T**alk **to y**ou **l**ater!

Acronyms

Work great for lists, both short and long. If you need a little extra help, you can use the first couple letters of a word, keep a word or two, or add a word or two! There are no true rules to follow. The purpose is to remember words! It doesn't matter how you do it. Just do what it takes to remember what you want!

Examples:
- Chop: **ch**eese, **o**nions, **p**otatoes
- Champ: **c**offee, **ham**burgers, **p**asta
- Pens: **p**aper, **e**nvelopes, **n**otebook, **s**tamps
- Gap bag: **ga**s, **p**ost office, **ba**nk, **g**roceries
- Solid: **so**ap, **li**ght bulbs, **d**ish detergent

Although the above acronyms are brief, they could be used for one trip to the grocery store and other errands. It's easier to remember five words over seventeen items! You will probably need to repeat the words with the letters then the acronym several times before you can remember them.

Teach

When you want to remember something with a lot of detail, teaching is ideal. Teachers have to be prepared in advance so they *write* notes, *study*, and *memorize* their lessons. Therefore, teaching can help you the same way.

- **Write notes** *Take notes* to gather all the information for your "lesson plan" or simply rewrite the information you need to remember. When you *write* notes, you are thinking intently.

- **Study** When you have all your information in front of you, study it as though you're preparing to teach it to someone else.
- **Practice memorizing** After you write *all* the information at least once and study it, practice memorizing it *one sentence or item at a time* until you can recite it without looking at your notes.
- **Teach** Once you've memorized everything, *teach it to another person or imaginary class/audience* if you must! Teaching always reinforces your memory because you have to learn, memorize, verbalize, and hear it again.

When you use all four steps together, you're reinforcing your memory as you make your brain review the same material by using four techniques. You can practice the same four steps for the same information as often as you like. The more often you exercise the techniques, the more likely you'll remember most, if not all of the information.

You're basically using a repetitious theme except with more depth. Just four easy steps and you're reinforcing and strengthening your memory.

Substitute Words (*a.k.a.*) Linking Words

Although the concept of "substitute" or "linking" words is typically used in English grammar to connect sentences, it can also work very well as a memory technique. When a word or name is hard to remember, you can break it up into syllables and turn the sounds of the syllables into different (substitute) words. You "link" or connect the "substitute" word with the original words and you'll have a memorable moment! You'll remember the words! This concept may seem complicated but it's not, it's actually fun!

Uncommon Unusual Words

Uncommon words are hard to remember because they don't "fit" into our everyday language. That's where "substitute" words come in handy. To remember words that are outrageously unique, linking them with other familiar words can make uncommon words really fun to remember. In order to remember them, you need words that make sense to you. And if possible, use words you'll be able to visualize. For example, the word telemetry sounds somewhat like, *tall lemon tree*! The words don't have to sound exactly the same or have any significance to the meaning. The trick is to simply link the substitute words and images to trigger the actual word you're attempting to remember. I use this technique regularly because it's fun and *works every time*!

NAMES

Just about everyone struggles with remembering names. "I'm terrible with names." is almost a cliché. But all it takes is at least one technique with some practice!

Use the Alphabet!

For people you know well but their name will not surface, go through the alphabet! You surely tried to remember something at one time in your life and the only thing you could remember is "it starts with," then you'd mention the particular letter it starts with. Before you know it, you remember the word! Your brain is capable of performing the same logic in reverse!

Personality and Features

- First and foremost get their name! Too often, we fail to register and hear the other person's name. How can you remember a name when you've never truly heard it!
- Don't worry about your appearance, shaking their hand, or anything else. Concentrate on paying attention to their name!
- Repeat their name back to them to assure you heard it right.
- As you talk to the person, address them by using their name throughout the conversation.

- Look into their eyes. Don't look around the room. You can't remember someone if you rarely look at them.
- Study them.
  - ► Use people associations. Compare the person with someone you're familiar with the same name *who:*
    - ► has a similar personality
    - ► has similar features
    - ► dresses the same way

Don't limit yourself. You can use friends, family, and even a public figure such as a celebrity! Anyone and any way will do! It doesn't matter which technique you use, as long as you use at least one memorable connection.

Tough Unusual Names

Use "substitute words." For example, to remember a last name like Baneski, you can easily use the words *"ban a ski."* The substitute words don't have to make sense. As a matter of fact, silliness works best! Substitute words are simply "triggers." Each time you use the substitute words, picture the person within the situation! For example, the substitute words for Baneski are ban - a - ski. Picture an angry person who's been banned from wearing a ski. They're mad because they can only wear one! Yes it's silly and even weird but it works. Try it!

NUMBERS

Most people have trouble remembering numbers. Our brains in general are notorious for lacking ability to remember numbers easily. Contrary to words that can be associated with an object, numbers are difficult to remember because they're abstract. Therefore, it's not an issue that only people with epilepsy struggle with it's a typical human issue! Just because remembering numbers appears to be an obstacle doesn't mean it can't be tackled.

Block it!

If you struggle remembering the date, use a daily "block" calendar. You'll change the number blocks daily which gives you two advantages. You need to physically turn the block(s) which causes you to concentrate and see the date intently. Using this simple procedure causes you to focus. If you just look at a calendar, you typically just glance at it. A brief glance may not be good enough.

Chunking
(Remembering numbers in groups)

Actually, this philosophy is not new to you! You've been "chunking" ever since you memorized your first phone number! Telephone numbers are broken into three "chunks" for practical purposes. After all, it would be very hard to remember a phone number which would look like this 6484354778. But since phone numbers are "chunked" 648-435-4778, they're obviously easier to remember! The same goes for social security numbers. It would take a lot to remember 154338240 but when it's chunked like 154-33-8240 it's almost effortless!

The beauty is, you can choose how many numbers you want in a "chunk!" The bad part is, you have to remember the numbers before you can chunk them! As far as *phone numbers* are concerned, there are two easy ways to remember them, connect them to special dates, like birthdays, anniversaries, and holidays or make them into other words that rhyme with the numbers.

With local numbers you usually only need to remember the last four digits. That makes it more fun and sometimes easier because you can turn the numbers into words! For example, the last four numbers are 9527. You can translate that into, nine lives to heaven! I honestly just typed in four numbers with nothing in mind. It's not hard and definitely fun.

Shape Up!

When you find it hard to remember a phone number, try using shapes or symbols. Look at the "face" of the keypad. Is there a pattern in the phone number that reveals a shape or symbol such as an arrow, square or X? For example, if the last four numbers are 7412, you'll see an arrow, 5689 you'll see a square, 1379 can be a Z!

Back to the ABC's

Many businesses use their name to help you remember their phone number. Even though you're trying to remember a personal phone number, you can still use the same concept. You just need to do it in reverse! Look at the letters on each button of the numbers in the correct dialing order. Then try to find a word that connects the number to the person or place.

Ideas to get you started, try the following to spell out the phone number:
- Their first name
- Nick name
- Last name
- Pet's name
- Workplace
- Street name
- Visualization and association (their hair or car color)!
- If you need to fill in a number or two, get silly by adding how you rate the person such as one is bad, ten is great, etc.

Yes, I'm stretching it but that's the point. It doesn't matter how you do it, just as long as it works! There's definitely no system to follow. Just make it memorable!

Visualization and Association

To connect information with your memory bank, the images must be memorable by making them drastically outrageous, impossible, and/or silly. It's the things that are out of norm that we tend to remember best. For example, I was invited to a special event while I was in a grocery store. I chose to use vivid images along with rhymes to remember the date. That was two years ago and I still remember the details!

The event was on the twentieth of June. I looked around for an easy way to connect with my worst memory enemy . . . numbers! But actually, with a little thought it came easy. I remembered *twenty* because there was "plenty" of food, and *June* because I wanted to get through the checkout "*soon!*" Seems silly but it worked and continues to stick in my memory! As far as numbers are concerned, this is by far the easiest memory technique that works for me.

Special Memories

For special moments, have family and friends remind you occasionally by simply saying something like, "Do you remember when . .?" When they do that over a few days or even weeks from each other, the mental picture and memory stays! I can remember a special event with my grandson, Gabe which took place five years ago, when he was only two years old. My neighbor, Gyasi was there. He reminded me of that special moment at least ten times over a month's period simply by saying, "Remember when Gabe pulled on your arm so you would bend down, and then he kissed you!" The beauty is, I don't only remember it but I can picture it as if it was yesterday!

Since it's such a workable "system," I taught my grandchildren, *Alleigh, Kaylee, Gabe*, and *Ayden* all at a young age of three! I'm looking forward to teaching my new grand daughter, *Kalbri!*

Practice!

Now that you have a head start, practice all the techniques you like best and fit your needs. Start around the house and practice with anything that connects with your preferred techniques. But don't stop there. When you're in the car, practice the chosen techniques as you drive down the road in the city, country, or suburbs! No matter where you are, there are plenty of places to practice. Never tire from practicing. The more you work on the ideal techniques, the better you'll get, and the more natural they'll come when in need.

As you can see, mentally remembering information almost always takes repetition along with a few techniques. Whatever technique(s) you choose, make it fun and enjoy remembering the bits and pieces of your life!

True Stories

I can remember things from long ago, but I have a horrible memory with things in the present. I cannot remember people's names, places I have visited, and so on. I am a legal assistant with a law firm. You have to have a good memory. There are so many things that can go wrong with this. My bosses will tell me to do something and I say, yes sir and then when they walk off, I am like, now what did they say? I have to go back and say sir? I have tried to keep a pad next to me, but by the time they are done saying what they say, I have forgotten to get the pad. It is so stressful.

At home I have a horrible time also. Remembering play dates, school functions, field trips, with the girls, plays, household chores that they are supposed to do, is difficult also. I really have a problem. Sometimes I feel as though they are taking advantage of my problem. My fiancé thinks so also. He gets onto them. I do too! So what do you do about that? I get so frustrated and my youngest has admitted that only ONE time has she used it to get her way. Probably more than that, but she only admitted to that one time. I see people that I KNOW but I cannot tell you who they are. They look so familiar and I know that I know their names, but I can't remember. People always tell me that I am getting old. I'm only 38 years old. I'm not old, but sometimes it sure feels like it. *C. Anderson, Monroe LA*

I hate not being able to remember things. It really stinks when it comes to school work. But I use tricks to remember things. I play around with words that are crazy. I hate Science because the words are so big, stupid, and unnecessary for everyday life but I have to learn them. So I make up words that sound like the dumb word I have to know and it works a lot. The hard part is remembering the definition! But at least I win half the battle, which is enough for me to pass the tests!
K. Walker, Lincoln NE

My memory has gotten really bad since the seizures have started. I have seizures in my memory lobe so that doesn't help me much either. I usually can't remember things I did last week. But I can remember things I did years ago but they are slowly fading away. It makes me think I am getting old and I have Alzheimer's or something. But I'm only 24 and other then seizures, as far as I know I am perfectly fine.

From what I know about the seizures I have is that anytime I try to remember something to do any kind of deep thinking, I go into a grand mal seizure then I am just damned if I do, and I'm damned if I don't. Sometimes I try to write stuff down so I remember them on like "post it" notes. That works sometimes but not always. I always lose things. I put something down then forget where I put them. My family just giggles at me and acts like it's not a big deal and the same with my boyfriend. They try to make me feel as if it's not a problem. The stress your body goes through because of seizures is horrible to be scared to live because you don't know when the next seizure is going to be is horrible.

I have one advice to any person with epilepsy out there trying to help with their memory problems. *Get post it notes*! Keep them everywhere in plain sight, get the nice bright ones, post them in the kitchen, at your computer desk, on your bedroom mirror, on your bedroom door, anywhere you can see them every day! If science can't fix the problem now, you'll find a way to get around it, my way at the moment is "post it!" Blessed be to all who have this problem.
J Murray, Norristown PA

I get so frustrated when my girl friend doesn't cut me a break when I have a problem with my memory. She does not seem to think that I should be just like everyone else that doesn't have epilepsy nor ever had brain surgery. I can't get her to realize that she could understand by going back in time and remembering how I used to be before I graduated from college. It was just a few months later when I started having seizures. I don't think my memory problem is as hard to deal with as her lack of understanding. It really hurts to hear her say, "Are you dumb or just toying with me?" It's not going to last if she continues to treat me like that. After all, I can't help it that my memory is so bad. But she can help it how she reacts to it. I guess it's up to her.
L. Singler, San Diego CA

I can never remember simple every day words when I'm just trying to carry on a conversation. I really mind it when I'm talking to someone I don't know. They look at me like I'm dumb or something. My family jokes around about it. Sometimes I laugh with them but sometimes it hurts. I guess it matters what mood I'm in. I hate forgetting things that are important to me like doctor's appointments, taking my medicine, and where I put something. I seriously think having a memory problem every day is as bad as having one seizure once a week. Maybe some people won't agree with that but being a college student makes it hard to deal with. Having a memory is really nice when you're in college!
A. Kingsley, Forest VA

I hate the way it takes so long to come up with a word. It doesn't matter whether it's in my head when I'm thinking about something or when I'm trying to talk. I can never remember where I put something. I try to remember on my own but no matter how hard I try, I never succeed. I have to make notes and put them all over my apartment. But sometimes I can't remember where I put them! The only thing I'm good at remembering is when to take my medicine because I do it the exact same time every day. That's one way I can remember something good, if it's something on a regular basis. But if not, I might as well be in the dark because that's what it's like.

D. Krepps, New York NY

The thing I hate about my memory problem is when I hear or see something and I try to recall it a minute or two later, it's gone. I can't remember any of it. I'll try really hard thinking it'll come back but it never does. The longer I deal with this, the more it aggravates me.

I hate being teased or yelled at for it. My parents think I should be like my brother and sister. I'm supposed to be "complete" but when it comes to letting me do the things they do, I'm different. I wish they'd make up their minds.

D. McKlanahan, Harrisburg PA

My memory has always been bad. I was diagnosed with epilepsy when I was eight years old. I don't remember a week without a seizure. My mom has helped me remember things by playing tricks with my mind! I have so many tricks to remember things that I forget the tricks! I'm kidding! Remembering things aren't always fun but I can do it when I try hard and use my tricks. I'm thankful my mom took the time to help me and most of all that she understands. I have a friend in school that doesn't have support from anyone but me. I taught her some of my memorizing tricks and she said it changed her life! I think that's so cool. I did something to change someone's life and all I did was teach her tricks!

B. Scott, Philadephia PA

My memory problem bothers me more than anything next to seizures. It's discouraging when people seem to think that since since seizures are almost controlled I shouldn't have any other side effects, especially a lack of memory. A friend of mine told me I was supposed to get over it and act normal. I was devastated. Needless to say, I broke off our friendship. I don't need friends like that. I want friends who are going to support me not drag me down worse than my memory problems. Little did I know that getting better control over seizures would not give me better control over my memory issues. I'm glad I'm seizure *free* but I wish I was memory deficient *free* also!
Tori, New York City NY

My biggest problem with epilepsy besides seizures, is the hard time I have coming up with words when I talk to people, especially when I'm talking to someone I don't know. It seems like the people look down on me, like I'm dumb. So I end up apologizing to them and explaining that I have epilepsy.
D. Pellock, Gainesville GA

I wish my doctor or his nurse would tell my dad that my memory problems are real. I told my doctor I'm having a hard time in school because I can't remember things. Instead of saying something, my dad jumped in and said I was just using that as an excuse because my grades are bad. The doctor never said it's normal for epileptics. He should at least tell him that so my dad won't get so discouraged and make me feel bad about something I can't help.
C. McGill, Smyrna GA

I do feel that my memory problems have caused just as much stress on me as the seizures. When I started having seizures (petit mals) in sixth grade, my memory was shot. School was so hard. I was always a good student, and then I had the hardest time getting though the day. I would study all night, get in class, and it would be gone. School became so hard. I worked so hard and finally got my grades up.

Two weeks before my graduation I found out I wasn't going to get to walk with my classmates. I missed my GA graduation test by one point. It was the science part. I couldn't for the life of me remember the periodic table. It made me so mad and hurt. I wanted to blame somebody and the only person was me! But now I know it wasn't me, it was the epilepsy. It hasn't only affected my school but my whole life.

I'm coming up on my five years seizure free which is big, but I still struggle everyday with my memory. It has affected my relationship with my boyfriend. It has become a big problem in our relationship. Where did I put this or when does this need to be done? I can't remember. It's so stressful and makes me feel like less of a person.

I am very hard headed, and when I think I'm right about where something is, it turns out that I'm wrong. It throws me down and it's a slap me in the face. It just reminds me how much epilepsy has and will always affect me. I write stuff down to help me remember but then I forget where I put it, so it doesn't help really.

I'm so scared that I will forget the first things my daughters do, their first steps, words, etc. I do write them down, and I have told others where it is. I feel as if I use it as an excuse sometimes but it's really not. It's the truth. I do wonder if my medicine is a part of my memory loss. It is a daily problem that I have to deal with and there isn't anything that can be done that I know of so I have accepted it. I don't like it but can't change it. It's just me!
Jessa, Dayton OH

I can't remember, I don't remember, etc. I say those words more often in a "daze" time than I used to in a total year before epilepsy.

I wonder if I should buy a T shirt that says, I don't remember! All kidding aside, it feels as if there's no help. I know there are a lot of people who are going through it too, but I still feel alone because my family doesn't understand. They get more annoyed with my quoting the infamous phrases than I do when from saying them. It's depressing.
Erika, Lansing MI

My little boy is learning to use my memory problem to his advantage. He's putting me in a position to try to find a solution to fixing it. But how do I remember everything that's said and done? Is that even plausible for anyone? My only means of staying sane is to tell myself it's the way it is, and feeling sorry for me isn't going to help. I try to look up to God and ask Him to help me cope and see it for the reason He's allowed it into my life.
M. Hardy, Alto CA

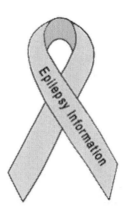

Epilepsy Friends

We all share common struggles with epilepsy. Therefore, getting around other people with epilepsy can offer consolation and a great deal of comfort and encouragement. There are many ways to make friends who have epilepsy but there's one way I strongly recommend. If you want to make friends, the best thing you can do is become proactive with epilepsy awareness, support, and advocacy.

If you long to feel loved, accepted, and respected, epilepsy advocacy is right for you. All you need to do is reach out to and for other people with epilepsy! I can assure you, everything you do will provide you with plenty of love, acceptance, respect, and friends. I promise that' you'll have fun, *if* you follow my suggestions! The time you invest will be well worth the benefits that you and your friends will receive. *The glory of friendship is not the outstretched hand nor kindly smile nor the joy of companionship. It is the spiritual inspiration that comes to them when they discover that someone else believes in them, understands their struggles, and is willing to trust them with their friendship.* That alone makes the job of advocacy inviting!

If you're not convinced you're needed within the epilepsy community, consider the following statistics seriously. One in 26 Americans will develop epilepsy in their lifetime. There are approximately

2.7 million people who have epilepsy in the United States alone. That averages out to one in a hundred people. When you do the math, it's obvious there are people around you who have epilepsy. It's also obvious that when someone is newly diagnosed, they need support from other people who truly understand their confusion, frustration, lack of understanding, and most of all support. They long to be helped, understood, loved indiscriminately, and more. The need is there, the people are there, and the irony is, they're just like you. All you have to do is bring everyone together into one big "family."

Let's consider you live in a small town like me with an approximate population of 600 people! And you think there are probably only four people who will join you at your events. To you, that may seem like a very small number and not worth all the energy you would put into it. But think out of the box. The four people you will be helping will have a positive influence on their families and friends through their improved attitude and self esteem. They may change enough to make a drastic change in everyone's lives. And the beauty is it might not stop there! They may help someone in another town get something started. Then their friends may start something in another town and on and on. Do you see what an impact *you* can make? One person can make an incredible change and touch a lot of lives with a little effort and a lot of love. If you're capable of sharing, loving, and helping others, you're capable of doing the job well.

Ways to Find Friends Who Have Epilepsy

Friends are indispensable because they're like angels, even though you can't see them, they're always there. It's no big secret that everyone feels more comfortable around people with whom they have a lot in common. Any function which reaches out to epilepsy friends can form a necessary bond. After all, we all seek love, help, and an avenue to vent our emotions. Don't hesitate to reach out to other people with epilepsy and be their best friend. The options mentioned in this section are by far not the only possibilities! There are surely more ways to befriend people with epilepsy. Go beyond my recommendations. Use or come up with some of your own!

Visit online epilepsy social websites. There are plenty of options. To find a site that suits your needs, search *epilepsy online social sites* and/or *seizure online social sites*.

Set up epilepsy information and support stands: Open an information stand at health fairs, local festivals, carnivals, community fairs, flea markets, etc. Most community events will provide the space at no cost to you since you're offering a community service. All you'll need is a table, at least three chairs, (one for you, your epilepsy friend, and their family member or friend), and epilepsy material. Contact your Epilepsy Foundation's local office for brochures. For free magazines. See: *Websites and Resources.* Refer to: *Epilepsy Magazines.*

Attend an annual "Epilepsy Family and Friends Support Day" picnic: If no such event exists in your area, I encourage you to start one. Again, you can make a difference in your community. It's sure to be a success. It's a great opportunity to make new friends, not to mention to help your loved ones.

The greatest advantage I found with the *Epilepsy Family and Friends Support Day* was sitting down in a relaxed fashion with other people who have epilepsy. It's so pleasantly comfortable talking about the things you have in common. I especially find it enjoyable when you're discussing similar situations and hearing you're new friend(s) say, "I know exactly what you mean! I do that too!" or "I always thought I was just weird." or "I'm so glad we talked about this." And it goes on and on! It's so refreshing to be able to sit down with other people and connect with them. After all, who else can you do that with!

And of course, your family and friends have a great time as they get together with other families and friends to discuss their common ground. And they'll enjoy seeing you at ease as you open up to others and make new friends. I can assure you, if you organize such an event, you'll have a great time. You'll make new friends and get refreshed!

Other great ideas for fellowship time with epilepsy family and friends, is to celebrate a major holiday. You can organize a Christmas party, Easter "e.e.g.," *(egg)* hunt, etc.!

No matter how you decide to bring everyone together, it can be done at no cost to you. If you need an indoor facility for something like a Christmas party, consider non-profit organizations such as the American Rescue workers, United Way, and Salvation Army. Please note all the previous organizations are autonomous therefore the same organization may have different fees if any. You can also contact the Information Referral Center for other options in your area. If you decide to plan a picnic, try to stay away from summer holiday weekends because people tend to get "burned out" from so much picnicking!

Free advertising options:
- Hang fliers in heavily traveled places such as; doctors offices, hospitals, grocery stores, banks, retail stores, convenience stores, gas stations, etc.
- News stations usually provide an online bulletin board for, "announcements and upcoming community events."
- Newspapers can give your event a lot of attention if you offer to share your story for an article, especially if you're sponsoring the first epilepsy event in your area.
- Radio stations are legally obligated to advertise for free on behalf of non profit community events!

Consider the following for a flyer layout:
- Title: Epilepsy Family and Friends Support Day picnic.
- Add place of event, date, and time.
- Make sure you accentuate "No charge."
- Contact event organizer for more details.
- Make pull off tabs on the flyers (include your first name and phone number).

The pull off tabs will make it easy for people to reply so you can organize the event. You'll be able to arrange who brings the necessary items such as drinks, cups, plates, etc. either with or instead of a covered dish.

Take index cards to the picnic so everyone can exchange their email addresses, phone numbers, etc. Be sure to supply a piece of paper for names, telephone numbers, addresses, and email addresses for yourself. That way you'll be able to contact them if you decide to have another event. You can also contact your local Epilepsy Foundation, and tell them how well it turned out. Invite them to join you for the next event. It would be advantageous to include them each year because they have so much to offer to you, your friends, and family. Once the Epilepsy Foundation is involved, they may decide to help organize each event.

If you'd like to have a picnic every year, it's a good idea to use the same weekend every time. That will make it easier for people to plan ahead. For example, schedule it for the third weekend of May.

Attend Epilepsy Foundation Events: You can help raise money for the Epilepsy Foundation through attending a "walk." All you have to do is contact your family, friends, and their family and friends for financial support. While you're walking, you will be getting exercise, earning money for the Epilepsy Foundation, and making new friends! If you'd like to take part in raising money for the Epilepsy Foundation and make new friends along the way, contact the Epilepsy Foundation affiliate nearest you. See: *Websites and Resources*. Request them to add you to their mailing list.

Attend or start a support group: You will most definitely receive benefits that will outweigh the distress you feel as you struggle on your own daily. Keep in mind, if you don't step out of your unpleasant little world, you might get stuck there. Get around the people that will truly be happy to help you grow and become a stronger person! If you won't do it for yourself, do it for the people you love. If you think, "I can't participate in a support group because I have too many seizures. I don't want to have seizures in front of anyone." Well, join the crowd! Join the crowd that knows and understands your hesitance. But it's time to step out and take a chance.

You need to be around friends who know what you're going through. Friends who feel the same way you do about having seizures in front of people. Go ahead, have a seizure in front of them. Believe it or not, it could be good for them! After all, how else can anyone understand what their family and friends see and feel? The best way to grasp what they're going through is to encounter and observe the same things they encounter and observe. You won't be causing your friends harm, you'll be helping them!

The bottom line is, you're not just supporting each other, you're supporting you're family and friends as well. You know all too well, you cannot truly understand another person's battle until you've experienced it yourself. The best thing you can do for your family and friends is see what they see. If you encounter a seizure during your time at a meeting, consider it an opportunity to better understand your loved ones and the emotions they feel. How can you expect them to love, understand, and accept your battle, when you won't even submit yourself to theirs?

On a different note, you need to be around other people within your circle. If you stay around people who have never suffered a seizure, you can't grow. You may be stuck thinking things such as, "I'm not good enough . . . "It's never going to get better," and/or "I'm nothing but a burden to my family and friends, etc." You probably won't walk with your head held high, when you're mostly around people who mock, tease, belittle, and/or fear you.

When you meet with your epilepsy friends, you can be taken out of that negative world and uplifted by others who know and understand your feelings because they feel them, too! You need to be with people who say, "I know exactly what you mean! I feel that way, too!" You will be amongst people who will be happy to lift you up on a regular basis. It's one of the best things you can do for yourself and your loved ones. You will truly know what it's like to completely enjoy integrity, peace, and respect. You can become an all around new person, and you'll no longer feel alone.

Digging Deep into the Hearts of Our Friends with Epilepsy

Can you relate to the following comments and concerns? Would you feel a sense of relief having conversations with people who have similar concerns? If your answer is yes, you would benefit greatly by attending or leading a support group and other epilepsy events. You may also be a great advocate to get something else started in your area. Consider it!

Lead a support group: Support groups have more than one purpose. Yes, everyone needs to talk about what's happening in their lives but its equally important to "brain storm" *pun intended*, to find answers to their issues. Open up the meeting with a thought provoking question or start with a theme. For example, you can ask something like, "What do you wish you knew from the beginning of your battle with epilepsy?" I asked that question on an online epilepsy social site. They responded with the following comments:

I wish I knew how many people really have epilepsy. I was alone but didn't have to be.
Jimmy J. New York, NY

There's far too many, but I think the biggest one is I wish I knew epileptologists existed. That would have made such a huge impact on my outcome. I also wish I knew the Epilepsy Foundation existed and all the available tests so I could have been properly treated from the beginning.
Diane

I wish I knew the Epilepsy Foundation existed!
Laura, G. Lansing MI

If I had known about the Epilepsy USA magazine, things could have been a lot easier.
Kayla G, Dallas TX

I wish I knew how involved and complicated epilepsy can be, and at the same time, so simple. I wish I was more of a self advocate in the beginning. I think that would have helped me get well sooner. I also wish I had done research. It is amazing how many tributaries run from the river of epilepsy. Treatments are so personalized.

I wish I knew to keep a journal from day one of symptoms, seizures, etc. You could look back and get a general idea of what is going on. I wish I knew there were so many different types of epilepsy, like catamenial, etc.

After my vagus nerve stimulator was implanted they told me that in a few days you will be okay. But in actuality, it takes at least a week or so. Every time you move your head, you use your neck and upper body where an incision is made and it is sore!
S. Lenon, Brighwood OR

I wish I knew how common epilepsy is, and that it is not just a mysterious disorder that is practically unheard of. Granted, many people in my life were unfamiliar with the disorder. But people would be surprised how many more people I have met that also have epilepsy. And how much mentioning it has brought us together. It's not something to be ashamed of it is something that makes us unique. Knowing that and getting to know other people with the disorder, has really made me feel like part of a community.
A. Faure, Valley Stream NY

I wish I knew how mine started. It was either by a fall on the back of a doll stroller when my aunt was babysitting me or a high fever or the German measles. They still don't know why. Plus it started right when I had my period when I was 8 ½ years old. Even when I had cancer and had my uterus and ovaries removed, I kept having them. They even thought it was a female thing. Even after 48 years they have gotten worse.

C. Flowers, Carmichael CA

I wish I'd known about epilepsy, and about people who are epilepsy advocates. I wish I knew about all of the useful information available in the various internet epilepsy groups. I can honestly say that I learned about Keppra before my first neurologist (he was not an epileptologist.) I also learned about SPM 927 (now named Lacosimide) before my current epileptologist. It got him back in gear, and he's sharp as a tack now! I wish I knew that you often have to be aggressive with some neurologists to get them to be really helpful. I'm sure you've found this to be the case, also.

W. J. Hurren, Fort Worth TX

I wish I could make people understand some stuff about epilepsy. One of the problems I have is everyone seems to want to "fix" me! For example, a friend told me she knows someone who just had an implant and it "fixed" her! I'm sure she was talking about the vagus nerve stimulator. They act like I've never read up on this stuff! They don't understand that every case and every person is different and there are different types of seizures. Then, she makes this "great discovery" that she's sure I've never heard about. The infamous seizure dog!

I had to explain to her that I don't need one. I know when I'm going to have a seizure! I don't need a dog to tell me how I feel! I'm sure they are helpful to some people but with different types of seizures. I went without insurance for a long time, and I just couldn't get the help I needed. I've had insurance for a couple years now, and I'm lucky enough to have found a great neurologist. I've been seizure

free for about eight months now! When and if I have another seizure, I'll rely on him to "fix" me!
B. Cunningham, Gastonia NC

As you can see, that simple question can open a lot of con- versation.

An opportunity to Share Your Personal Stories

Getting something started or attending events with other people who have epilepsy doesn't mean you have to sit around in "gloom and doom." After all, epilepsy isn't all gloom and doom. There are plenty of ups and downs. The downs don't have to be the majority of conversation during a meeting. You can enjoy each others "ups!" However, no matter how enjoyable you want the meetings to be, it's important to allow everyone to vent their emotions and struggles.

No matter which way the meeting goes, you can always end it with a pleasant tone. Be prepared to share something positive so everyone will go home feeling better and prepared to take on their world. For instance share about a new treatment in research. The following stories are a sample of what you might hear during a meeting.

I was 21 when I was at a college football game with my girlfriend. I was standing in line to buy drinks and French fries and had a grand mal seizure. Someone found a campus cop to help me. I couldn't believe his reaction. He harassed me! He insisted I was drunk! I insisted I wasn't and that he needed to call my girlfriend on her cell phone. He did the same thing to her. He insisted I was drunk and that she shouldn't try to cover up for me because she could get in trouble, too! He was trying to intimidate her into admitting I was drunk!

People were gawking at me like I was a criminal. I have never been in trouble with the law! Not only was I not drunk, I've never drank an alcoholic beverage my entire life! To be accused of being drunk was really humiliating. It made it obvious that people with epilepsy are misunderstood and people are uneducated. But for a cop to be uneducated is insulting.

I saw that officer a few weeks later and confronted him about how he handled the situation. He apologized to me! He admitted he was uneducated about epilepsy. He said he was telling another cop what happened and it turned out, he had epilepsy, too! The other cop told him he probably made a big mistake and that it was unlikely I was drunk. He told him, it's extremely unlikely that anyone would use epilepsy and seizures to cover up being drunk! So the cop apologized to me again! He said he'd learn more about epilepsy and teach his peers.

I've been wearing an epilepsy medical alert bracelet ever since! I'm determined to never let that happen, again! Once is enough! I also started teaching my friends more about epilepsy. Every time I get an opportunity, I teach people! I guess in a way I became an advocate!
J. Reighard, Daytona Beach FL

The seizures I have are controlled by two medications but that was after several unsuccessful attempts with four medications prior to the ones I am currently taking. Supposedly my neurologist is one of the best in the business. But isn't it odd that after a recent stay in the hospital and being referred to a psychiatrist, she was the one who figured out what the heck was wrong with me?

My neurologist is one of those doctors who seem to be too busy to really get to know you. And she likes to push medicine. I was recently married. It's been about a month now and I'm on a different insurance, so it's forcing me to change neurologists. I'm on the search for a new one with the mindset that another opinion really won't hurt anything! It's great to talk to someone who has a clue what I am talking about and going through!
Renee, Natrona Heights PA

I'm 43 years old, and I had epilepsy most of my life. When I was first diagnosed, I was 11 years old. That was when I was told by a specialist that I probably had epilepsy. First, second, and third grade were years I don't remember real well. I would glare into space and was not able to answer the teacher. At that time, they did not know I was having seizures so they would punish me. Then I would get punished at home. Because of this, I did not get my education like most people. But I finally graduated!

I was supposed to graduate in 1982 but instead, I graduated in 1984! I still have epilepsy but now it is better controlled. I only have seizures in my sleep. I've been employed for seven years! I would like to thank you for having this Myspace for a person with epilepsy. I have always been afraid of speaking out to other people about my epilepsy.
K. Charles, Danville KY

I have epilepsy as a result of a condition called Sturge-Weber Syndrome. I've had seizures my whole life. Before 1997, the worst thing to ever happen was a broken index finger and a cut on my chin that required stitches. On Thanksgiving Day 1997, everything went downhill. The seizures usually begin after several days of suffering from a migraine headache. I made it to my mother's for dinner that day. I was still in a great deal of pain. When we got to my mom's, I laid down on the couch. That is the last thing I remember until Saturday evening. I began having uncontrollable seizures. I was rushed to a local hospital where I was then taken by helicopter to a hospital in Dayton, OH.

That's where we found out the seizures had shut my kidneys down. I had to be put on dialysis. There is nothing worse than having your liquid intake rationed! My kidneys weren't functioning so everything I drank stayed in me. I was like a balloon. At one point I was so desperate for a Mountain Dew that my brothers brought one in! The nurse let me drink it and then sucked it back out! Anyway, Sunday afternoon I woke up, and a doctor was putting a tube in my chest.

I had a total of six treatments and my kidney function returned! The doctor came and removed the catheter after the last treatment. They said kidneys don't usually shut down often. Now I have a scar on my chest to remind me to never take anything for granted.
D. Bones

Yes, it was unfortunate that I was not breathing when I was born; I'm guessing a bad c-section. I have problems because of it. But I'd rather be proactive in who I am and what I do.
Shelly

Ideas to Close a Meeting

Encourage members to discuss issues that are causing personal problems. Have a member share something that's encouraging. Attempt to include most or all of the members in the discussion to develop a sense of family. Present great information such as success stories from epilepsy magazines and websites. Update members about new studies.

Make sure you keep the meeting in an orderly fashion, always allowing members to share both good and bad. Attempt to work the issues out *together*. As the leader, enjoy having the last word. Simply leave them with an emotional strengthening thought-provoking quote to stimulate an over all feeling of well-being.

End of the Meeting Quotes

"No one can make you feel inferior without your permission." Eleanor Roosevelt

"Do what you can, with what you have, and where you are." Theodore Roosevelt

"Any fact facing us is not as important as our attitude toward it, for that determines success or failure." Norman Vincent Peale

"If you live your life afraid because you're afraid to live, then you live no life at all." Author Unknown

"Make up for your weaknesses by concentrating on your strengths." Diane Keeler

"What lies behind us and what lies before us are tiny matters compared to what lies within us." Oliver Wendell Holmes

"God gave us two ends. One to sit on and one to think with! Success depends on which one you use; heads you win – tails, you lose!" Author Unknown

"I think a hero is an ordinary individual who finds strength to persevere and endure in spite of overwhelming obstacles." Christopher Reeve

"Why not go out on a limb? Isn't that where the fruit is?" Frank Scully

"Your situation isn't your destination. It's meant to be your motivation." Author Unknown

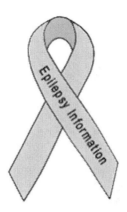

Seizure Resonse Dogs
A blessing & "best friend" all in one package!

Seizure response dogs are a special type of service dog, specifically trained to help someone with intractable epilepsy. Each dog goes through a specialized training. The initial training is for qualification. Then the dog goes through a second training with their potential owner in order to satisfy their specific needs. Labradors and Golden Retrievers are preferable "candidates" because of their natural interest in retrieving and pleasant temperament. That does not mean other dogs cannot be utilized, it simply means they are both known for successfully completing the trainings and fulfilling their "job" requirements.

The following poem was written by *S. Christoffer, Iowa City*

Amber is my name
Responding is my game
I never miss a day
I work hard for my pay
Give me your love and devotion
I will sleep with one eye open
I went to school and got an education
Therefore, I know what is best for your situation
With every year that we grow older
I take the weight of disability off your shoulders
I am here to please so I am eager
To help you when you have a seizure
Public servants interfere and take me from my job
While my partner is helpless and lays there and sobs
They stand above my partner and smirk
Let me go and get back to work
I can help, for you would not know
For you cannot get past your big ego
You may say, "Only Guide Dogs Allowed"
Modify your policies and get with the crowd
Your narrow minds think I am in the way
Maybe, just maybe, you will get it someday
You walk around as if it will not affect you
You could end up in my partner's shoes
Society may think of her as a menace
But with me by her side
She achieves independence
I am a seizure response dog
Do not pet me. I am working!

The following questions were answered by the seizure response dog organization, *Paws with a Cause:*

What is the process for acceptance into the program? An application must be filled out.

Is there an age requirement? The minimum age to receive a PAWS Seizure Response Dog is 14 years old.

What are the requirements to receive a dog? The individual must experience seizures on a regular basis; at least twice per month on average.

What is the usual expense from beginning to end? Currently there is no expense to the client until the dog is placed. Once placement occurs, the client is responsible for the dog's care, including food, grooming, veterinary care, etc.

How long does a typical training take? Seizure response dogs are trained at our facility for four to seven months. This is followed by approximately six months of work in the home with the team, facilitated by a local representative.

What does training involve? Training involves obedience and tasks specific to the needs of the client, depending on the type of seizure(s) and their environment. This can include the dog being trained to get help from a person in the area, activating a life-alert system, blocking/ bracing, etc.

Do you train a dog who is already established with their owner? We will consider a client's own dog however it rarely works out successfully, due to many variables, such as the dog's age, our medical and temperament testing requirements, and the dog needing to train at our facility for approximately six months.

Is there a federal law in which state laws must follow? The Americans with Disabilities Act (ADA) contains provisions for assistance animals. However, each state has its own law in this regard.

Is it media hype that the dogs are trained for detecting seizures? We believe the answer is yes. We have documentation on only thirteen of over 150 PAWS seizure response dogs that have developed the detection behavior reliably. This was something the dogs developed on their own, *after* bonding for a significant amount of time with their partner. It cannot be guaranteed to happen. We do not believe a dog can be trained for this task, and have not seen documentation of the claim otherwise.

Your assistance dog will:
- Provide physical and emotional support.
- Either summon for help, by activating a medical alert on a pre pro-grammed phone or find another person to assist you.
- Block individuals who have absence seizures from walking into streets or other possible dangerous places as well as prevent them from walking into harmful obstacles.
- Be able to pull potentially dangerous objects away from you.
- Carry information regarding your condition.
- Attempt to arouse you from unconsciousness *after* a seizure.
- Retrieve a phone for you, prior to a seizure.
- Stay with you during a seizure.
- Instill confidence.
- Provide companionship and contribute to your overall emotional well-being.
- Be your best friend!

Over several years of ownership, some dogs may develop a natural ability to sense an impending seizure, which will then urge them to alert you of your impending danger. However, this is an *uncommon phenomenon*. It should not be an expected trait by any dog whether trained or untrained. Some untrained dogs may help their owners, although there are reports that many have reacted aggressively. Some have even died due to witnessing or anticipat-ing their owner's seizure. The news media has provided a grave disservice by misleading the public that a good part of the serv-ice provided by seizure response dogs is to alert their owner of an oncoming seizure. Unfortunately, that is a fallacy. A dog cannot be trained to detect seizures. It is strictly a phenomenon that the dog is naturally gifted.

Seizure response dogs must be capable of maintaining control in every possible situation. A training facility reported they tested 385 dogs and 107 puppies. Only ten had the qualities they were looking for in a seizure response dog. Due to the difficulty in training and the limited resources of dogs, only a few organizations provide seizure response dogs. However, the numbers are rising.

To sum it up, the purpose of a seizure response dog is not to detect seizures but to protect you from injury, summon for help, and of course encourage independence. Seizure response dogs are licensed for medical reasons. Each state has its own set of laws within the guidelines of the "Americans with Disabilities Act." The laws protect you and your dog from discrimination.

Service dogs are generally allowed anywhere that the public is allowed. Privately owned businesses that serve the public, such as concert halls, hotels, restaurants, retail stores, sports facilities, taxicabs, buses, and theaters are prohibited from discriminating against individuals with disabilities. The *Americans with Disabilities Act* (ADA) requires all privately owned businesses to allow you and your dog, entrance onto their premises into all the areas customers are generally allowed.

If you go into a business, and are told your dog cannot go inside, simply inform them of your need for your dog. The business cannot insist you expose your disability, nor can it demand proof that your dog is certified as a service dog. However, it is wise to carry your dog's certification papers to avoid any hassle. In addition to the federal law, there are state laws that provide additional protection to service dogs and the people they serve.

How to handle a person who denies service dog entrance:
- Show an identification card.
- Explain that your dog is protected under the law used for guide dogs, for the blind through the Americans with Disabilities Act.
- Show your copy of the law.
- Ask to speak with the manager or supervisor, and repeat all the previous steps.

If the person still denies your dog from entering, Document the following:
- Date and time
- The person's name and title

- Name of business
- Address of business

Ask the person to sign a statement that you have explained the above. They will probably deny signing it however; it shows you are prepared to handle the situation. Consider yourself an educator. This may be their first time to see a service dog. You will probably make a new friend!

If you are still denied access with your dog, you should call the police. You most likely will need to educate the police officer as well! Make sure to point out the federal violation, and that it is a criminal misdemeanor, therefore, comes under police enforcement. It is vital to document everything if you decide to press charges.

True Stories

I am still waiting for my seizure dog. It was a very long application process, pages upon pages. I had to write an autobiography and get doctors letters as well as proof from a social worker that I was an appropriate candidate. Then I underwent an interview over the phone before being approved. It has now been over a year. I was told the wait could be up to three years.

This would be the opportunity of a lifetime. I could leave my home and go out in the community. I could even be alone in my home! I could have "me" time! It is hard to be patient but when you have such an amazing chance, you have no choice.
K. Doyle, East Waterboro ME

My dog, Penny was not trained as a seizure dog. I got her when I was in my late teens when I was having tonic - clonic seizures about twice a week. She quickly learned to take care of me.

Fourteen years later when she was riddled with arthritis and could not climb stairs due to the pain; I had a seizure (the first in years). I

was upstairs in a house that was not seizure proof. I cut myself so badly that I certainly would have died. Penny climbed the stairs and licked my face until I was awake enough to call for help. My dog did not have any formal training but she learned quickly that I needed help, and she could help me. This was what she did last.
D. Colera, Santa Monica CA

As a child, I was diagnosed with petit mal epilepsy. Once I hit puberty, the diagnosis was reversed, and I was told I was epilepsy free! For the following 14 years, I carried on like a person without a seizure condition; driving, attending parties, and concerts with strobe lights, regular unsupervised swimming, etc. On June 29, 2005, I offered a friend a ride to work, and brought my dog, Cosmo along for the drive. Moments after entering the freeway, Cosmo started to bark and cry uncontrollably.

My friend looked over at me to notice that I was frozen and in the grips of my first adult seizure. He managed to gain control over the vehicle from the passenger seat, veer to the exit ramp, and contact an ambulance. Weeks later, I was diagnosed again with epilepsy. I am happy to say that I have not had a seizure since, that I am aware. However, I have given up driving entirely.

This is a reward for my dog for saving my life. We take twice as many walks now. However, this is not necessarily a story about a trained seizure response dog, my medically untrained Cosmo proved to me that day that he was my seizure response dog. Without his barking and crying, my friend may not have been aware of the seizure that I was having, and may not have had the opportunity to gain control of the car before being involved in an accident.
D. Lyons, New Orleans LA

I had a golden retriever, Chahncy who would sense a seizure coming on. He would push my kids Torri, Rikki, and Lexxi away from me when I was going to have a seizure. Then he would lay on me until I got up. He did that for about six or seven times. I also had a Saint Bernard and a sheep dog but Chahncy was the only one who tried to help me.

Scott, Riverhead NY

My reply is not about a seizure response dog exactly but rather a dog that responds to seizures. Hunter is just a mutt with no training at all. Back when I had grand mals (generalized tonic-clonic) more frequently before my last brain surgery, I would find Hunter lay at my side when I woke up. I sometimes noticed him acting excited before I seized. This made me consider getting a younger dog that could be trained to be a seizure response dog. In fact, we purchased a standard schnauzer for that purpose.

W. J. Hurren, Ft. Worth TX

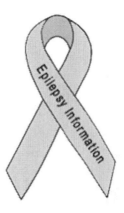

Parenting Your Child with Epilepsy

Raising a child with epilepsy is certainly not easy, and it will almost certainly change your life. Children are viewed as delicate little people who are easily harmed by the world. That is true to a degree but they won't be able to learn how to protect themselves from the world unless you teach them to be aware of their own dangers.

Small children already have typical dangers to learn about, yet alone having to deal with the threat of seizures. However, if appropriately supervised, an elementary age child is capable of safely living within their environment with the assumption their environment has been made seizure friendly.

Just because your little one has epilepsy doesn't mean they aren't capable of learning how to look out for themselves. Especially if you teach them as well as allow them, to get minor injuries to learn from. Yes, it's difficult since it's your nature to protect your child. However, over protection is not good for them because it can stunt them from growing up one step at a time.

Since all children are not created equal, do not be quick to compare your child with other children who have epilepsy.

Household safety is a crucial issue. The bathroom and kitchen are two of the most hazardous rooms in your home. You need to take extra precaution to prevent serious accidents. Your child should never take a bath alone regardless of their age. When they are old enough to bathe alone, they should only take a shower.

The kitchen is a threat to all young children for serious burns however your child is more susceptible to injuries. Staircases are also a threat to your child. Be sure to keep a gate at the top of each staircase. When your child needs to go up or down, they should not do so without your supervision. See: *Coping with Epilepsy.* Refer to: *Seizure Proof Your Home.*

As your child grows up and notices they're being protected more than other children their age, they may start to feel uncomfortably different. If that occurs, teach your child that feeling "different" is something many children experience in one way or another. For example, if other children have freckles and/or wear glasses they'll feel and be treated different even by other children. Teach your precious little one that when they're different that means they're special!

You must go the extra mile to balance their need to be independent along with the need to keep them safe. They should be encouraged to participate in safe activities they enjoy, yet help them understand the reality of the dangers you are protecting them from. This will help them understand you're not restricting them because they are wrong but protecting them because they are loved!

Siblings may feel a sense of resentment towards your child with epilepsy due to the amount of attention they are receiving from you. Some siblings might feel at fault or fear they'll get seizures, too. So it's up to you to provide an opportunity for them to vent their feelings. It's important for you to demonstrate and reinforce attention and caring feelings towards all your children.

Since such a demand can be difficult to fulfill, request family members and/or friends to allow you "time off" so you can take, one child at a time on a "date" once in a while. You can go to the movies, the park, or where ever *they* choose. This will give them a sense they are just as special. While you're on the date, don't bring up anything about your child with epilepsy. Only discuss them if your child brings them up. Even then, let them control the length of the conversation. Be sure to be open and honest. Most children know when they're being deceived. Be sure to provide them an opportunity to ask questions or address all their fears. But most importantly, do whatever you can to make the "date" special for them.

Raising Your Teen

About 400,000 children in the United States alone have epilepsy, and most of them are able to control the seizures and lead normal lives. However, as you know, epilepsy is a difficult task to manage.

As their parent, you will have to make sure your teen is taking their medications. It's important to let them take responsibility for taking them accurately and on time while keeping a keen eye to be sure they do so properly. You'll also need to teach them how to avoid their seizure triggers. It's tempting for teens to do what their peers do. So be sure they realize the dangers and how important it is to be especially careful in avoiding their triggers.

One of the most difficult issues to manage in the teen years is self-esteem. All teens are subject to plummet at one point or another during those delicate years. However, there are ways to help prevent serious struggles with self-esteem. See: *Living with Epilepsy in the Teen Years*

It may become a necessity to become an advocate for your teen. You may need to educate their teachers, school officials, your family and their friends. People who do not understand epilepsy may be frightened off and/or feel indifferent towards your child and their delicate condition.

The teen years can be a huge struggle for you, especially allowing your teen to become independent. It's only natural to want to protect your child. There's nothing wrong with that, after all it's your job as a parent. However, over protection can cause them problems.

Instead of trying to protect them from getting hurt, work on teaching them to handle situations and to deal with anything harsh that may come their way. Once your child becomes a teen, it's time to allow freedoms so they can gradually join the adult world. In order to accomplish this goal, you need to exercise flexibility. The most desired mission for teens is to establish independence.

You don't have to fear allowing them to establish independence. After all, you are not going to shove them into the world with no skills. You're going to start one step at a time.

Steps to Help Your Teen Earn Independence:
- Teach them the people who mind, don't matter, and people who matter, don't mind! It's as simple as that!
- Exercise your own strength because that will encourage them to be strong, as well.
- Help them improve their ability to make important decisions for themselves.
- Help them open up to their peers. See: *Living with Epilepsy in the Teen Years.* Refer to: *Telling people you have epilepsy.*
- Assist them in recognizing their identity. Make sure they know without a doubt that epilepsy is what they have not who they are.
- Build up their self-esteem. Studies show that parents have the greatest influence on their child's self esteem.
- Encourage them to find a job. As long as you allow them to find the job, it will help them feel a sense of adulthood and independence.
- Encourage them to think toward their future's plans.

Just like other students, they can get information from counselors, teachers, parents, and some extra help from the Epilepsy Foundation. But the most important step is that they do the "foot work" and make the decision on their own.

When adults with epilepsy look back on the challenges they faced as teens, many say it was not the epilepsy itself that caused the most obstacles but rather how their families and friends dealt with it. So it's important for you to achieve a balance. You are a very important tool in helping them. If you step out of your "comfort zone" and help your child live the closest teen life as possible, compared to that of other teens, they will be able to look back from adulthood and say, "I'm so thankful my parents were strong enough to let me live my life! I know it was tough but they loved me enough!"

If you still think letting go is too difficult, think of a mother bird. She protects her young but when the time comes, she gets them to spread their wings as she pushes them out of her nest! She knows there are animals which can harm them but it's her nature to nudge them so they'll take on the world independently. As hard as it is for you, it's also your job to get your child to spread their wings and take on the world. They'll be okay. They'll surely suffer difficult moments but we all do. That doesn't have to be a bad thing! Difficult times make most people stronger. You can prove your love to your child as you step aside and let them spread their wings. Allow them to grow strong so they can independently face the world around them.

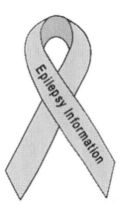

Living with Epilepsy in the Teen Years

Being a teenager is tough. As you know, being a teenager with epilepsy can be even tougher yet. But it's something that can be worked out. That doesn't mean epilepsy won't promote struggles and obstacles but there are ways to work around them to make life a little easier and more enjoyable.

Having the right perspective needs to be first on your list of priorities. If you believe your problem is so big that you will never see true happiness and it will never get better, you're hurting yourself more than the epilepsy itself. The bigger you see the epilepsy you struggle with, the more difficult it will be to deal with. In other words, your perspective makes a big difference in dealing with epilepsy.

You can and will succeed, *if* you have the right mindset and are determined and persistent regardless of your condition. Take note, I called epilepsy a condition which means, existing circumstance. Simply stated, epilepsy is a circumstance that can be worked through. It can be either big or small depending on your perception. Make it small so you can enjoy the best years of your life.

"Nothing can stop the man with the right mental attitude from achieving his goal; nothing on earth can help the man with the wrong mental attitude." W.W. Ziege

It's important to recognize that epilepsy doesn't define who you are, your personality does! Are you nothing but one big seizure? Of course not! Are you a person with feelings, desires, dreams, and plans? Of course you are! That means epilepsy is just an annoying fraction of your life. It's a health issue. Don't let it become a personality issue. Epilepsy is what you have, not who you are!

Epilepsy certainly shouldn't keep you from living out the best years of your life. Don't let it keep you from expanding yourself. Yes, you struggle with a lot of major issues but the very issues that are holding you back are the same issues that can make you a stronger, more determined, and more insightful person. Manage the epilepsy don't let the epilepsy manage you.

Sports and epilepsy do not have to collide. Epilepsy doesn't have to keep you from playing sports. Actually, participation in sports is usually encouraged by doctors. Even the most popular sports shouldn't present a problem. If playing a sport is a strong desire, go for it with your doctor's approval! But when you go for try outs, be sure you have someone near you who knows seizure first aid. No matter what sport you choose, be sure to tell your coach so he/she can learn seizure first aid and be ready to help you if a seizure occurs.

Tips for picking the right physical activities and sticking to them:
- You need to be comfortable wearing head gear when participating in a contact sport which involves a risk of falling or hitting your head.
- If the seizures usually occur around a certain time, plan the activities accordingly.
- Avoid extreme heat.
- Keep hydrated with plenty of *water* to reduce seizure risks.
- Do not drink anything with caffeine!
- Do not drink anything that's meant to give you energy.
- If you choose a sport in which you have to wear a helmet, be sure to have a lot of ventilation.

The following activities may need to be restricted, if you have uncontrolled seizures:

- Swimming
- Climbing to unsafe heights
- Riding a bicycle or motorcycle
- Skateboarding
- Horseback riding

I know it's not a particularly pleasant list but it keeps you safer. That's a sport you can always play, "play it safe!" All activities should be considered "off base" if, you want to do them alone.

Medication As a teen, medication can be very difficult to deal with. If the side effects are causing you to struggle, you should make an attempt to remedy the problem. There's obviously no such thing as the perfect medication because most cause some form of side effects. However, there's a possibility your medication may need a minor dosage adjustment and/or timing to help ease the effects. If your greatest problem is sleepiness, a medication adjustment may be significant enough to make a difference with the least potential for negative side effects.

It never hurts to check it out. Saying something to your doctor does not make you obligated to make any changes. However, it does offer you options. If you're on a medication that's working reasonably well, a little change in your medication schedule will be well worth checking into. The only way you will know if medication adjustments will be the answer to your problem, is to discuss it with your doctor.

Medications can cause unpleasant side effects even with the proper dosage and schedule. Since that may be the case, you may have an occasional desire to quit taking them. Maybe because the side effect(s) seem unruly or sometimes you're put in the position to explain why you take them or because taking them causes you to feel stigmatized. Each issue can be remedied which will help alleviate the stress. So it's important to deal with all of them now!

No matter what's causing you to dislike your medication, you must take it correctly! After all, if you don't take it correctly or simply do not take it at all, how much more explaining are you going to have to do to your friends, after you have a seizure in front of them? Try to think about your medication as helping you do things you want and need to do. It doesn't have to separate you from your friends or make you feel like an outcast.

Telling people you have epilepsy is a delicate matter. First, it's important to accept the fact you have epilepsy. If you came to terms with it, you won half the battle. Being honest with your friends and other people in your life is the next important step to take. You need to educate yourself so you'll have an upper hand on your struggles. You also need to educate others so they will have a better understanding to what epilepsy really is. That will be key to removing the fears and myths they may have. Remember the famous saying, "knowledge is power."

If it's something you want to run from because you know how hard it's going to be, keep in mind how equally important it is. Yes, telling your friends will be hard, so practice on your school nurse! She's safe because it's illegal for her to repeat your medical information to anyone else. So there's no room for her to gossip. She's also safe because she's a medical professional and is highly unlikely to shun or judge you. As a matter of fact, she'll probably be a great understanding friend. She may be able to guide you. Even if you haven't had a seizure in a long time, it's important to at least tell her. You're not obligated but if she knows beforehand, she'll be better prepared to help you in the event of a seizure. As you can see, you'll not only be helping yourself but also helping her.

You should not be intimidated nor feel embarrassed to tell your friends or anyone else about your condition. Remember, the *people who mind don't matter, and the people who matter don't mind!* That is a precious truth everyone with epilepsy should grasp. You should immediately reassure your friends you are just fine. Most of them will probably be surprised at first. But the more confident and calm you are, the easier it will be for them to accept and remain calm. With your assurance, they'll realize you're a teenager just like them who just happens to have epilepsy.

If you want to take the stress away from the personal seriousness of the subject, take this book with you when you tell them. You can ease the situation as you have fun with the comments in *A Different Look at Epilepsy,* and *Myths and Facts* chapters. That way you'll be educating and enjoying yourselves all at one time! Another option is to go to *Famous People with Epilepsy* so everyone can see how epilepsy does not stop people from achieving a full life.

Building your self-esteem is an important step in dealing with epilepsy. First of all, don't kid yourself into believing all "healthy" teens are happy and have good self-esteem. Everyone feels inferior sometimes. Everyone has something about themselves in which they dislike.

The following are ways to build or adjust your self esteem:
- Recognize you are not alone.
- Face epilepsy head on.
- Accept yourself as you are.
- Believe you are deserving of close friendships. An old proverb: *The best way to have a good friend is to be a good friend.* There's at least one "best" friend for everyone.
- Focus on the things that can be changed not on things that can not.
- When others attempt to belittle you, just shrug them off. "No one can make you feel inferior without your permission!" *Eleanor Roosevelt*
- Know without a doubt, you are worthy and deserving of love.
- Insist on respect. If you expect little, you'll receive little.

Puberty and menstruation can certainly affect some types of epilepsy. Research indicates there may be a relationship between changing seizure patterns and the onset of puberty. You may have experienced the first seizure within months of the time you began to have your period. Many girls who began to have seizures as children find their seizure types and patterns change with the onset of puberty. If you see a pattern with the seizure activity and menstruation, it's important to tell your doctor. Your treatment might need to be adjusted accordingly.

On a more positive note, if the seizures are influenced by your period, you might see a pattern which may work to your advantage. As you record your cycle and seizure activity precisely, you might find a pattern. If the seizures are mostly triggered by menstruation and your cycle is regular, it might be a benefit! With a dependable pattern, it might be easier to arrange activities. You could have the luxury of planning activities with your friends within your "safe" time, with less fear of having a seizure. It's surely not a guarantee but it can certainly be helpful.

Driving privileges are legal for people with epilepsy under certain circumstances. If the seizures are completely under control, there are no limits. Every state grants drivers licenses to people with epilepsy. But you must be seizure free for a period of time which varies from state to state. In most states, it will be necessary for your doctor to certify that you have been seizure free for the legal time limit.

I understand not having driving privileges and watching your friends get their licenses is almost unbearable. But try to accept the situation as temporary. Even though it hurts to watch your peers get their licenses, take note you're not the only teen who's not driving. Try to look at the situation as a temporary inconvenience while reminding yourself it's for your safety and the safety of others.

I know it's hard but if you look at it in the proper light it won't hurt so badly. Instead of feeling depressed, look forward to the future. You will drive some day! Instead of begrudging your present situation, try to save all your negative energy for when you finally get behind the wheel. After all, you will need a lot of energy to yell at the drivers who pull out in front of you, cut you off, and steal your parking spot, etc.!

The inability to attend school is no doubt very hard to deal with and accept. However, your teen years can still be enjoyable. You don't have to be kept from your friends. You can still be involved in extracurricular activities such as attending sporting events, hanging out at your friend's homes, and scoping the mall. You know what's safe and practical for your particular situation, so think it through.

There are definitely places to get together with your friends, in order to be the teenager you crave to be.

Dating can be a challenge for teenagers with epilepsy. But just because it's a challenge doesn't mean it's impossible. If you're dating someone now, you should be honest with them as soon as you feel comfortable talking to them about personal issues.

If you're going on a date, and the seizures are difficult to predict, you need to consider telling him/her upfront in case a seizure occurs while you're with them. In the world of epilepsy, the best way to look at it is, it's better to be safe than sorry. If you feel it's not safe to share the fact you have epilepsy with your date, find a new date! You don't want to get emotionally attached to someone with whom you feel won't be able to accept you because you have epilepsy. They need to see you as a person not as someone with epilepsy. In other words, they need to see you for who you are not for what you have.

If you're afraid to tell them you have epilepsy, then it's time you take a long look at yourself in the mirror, and give yourself a "pep" talk! You are just as good as everyone else. The minor flaw called epilepsy should not keep you from opening up to the people you like.

If you already have a boyfriend/girlfriend and you didn't tell them you have epilepsy, it's time to tell them. If you're afraid to tell them because you're afraid they'll break up with you, tell them anyway! After all, they're going to find out sooner or later! Don't be afraid to tell them. If they are so shallow that they'd break up with you because you have epilepsy, why do you want them? Granted, you're in love, but are they? If the ball was in the other court, and they had a serious health condition, would you break up with them?

The bottom line is it boils down to their character. If they really love you, nothing will interfere. With that in mind, you shouldn't be afraid to tell them you have epilepsy. After all, it's a great test of love! If they end up breaking up with you, they were undeserving of your love in the first place!

Education

Graduating from high school is something every mature teen desires. But for some with epilepsy it can be a hard task to achieve. Everyone with epilepsy has some level of trouble with their memory, which may cause complications in learning at a regular pace. See: *Memory Issues and Solutions,* Refer to: *Memory Techniques*

Going to school with your friends may be your most desired form of education. But if you're unable to attend, there are several options that can still provide you with an education that is acknowledged by both colleges and employers.

Home school is obviously learning at home. You can get the exact same books and all the other learning materials provided to students in public schools; because the school district is funded by taxes which obligates them by law whether you physically attend school or not.

Cyberschool is primarily a computer-based curriculum with account-ability methods through the internet. Every state has its own rules and regulations. In many states, it's paid through tax dollars with no cost to the parents.

G.E.D. Getting a G.E.D. may not be the answer to your heart's desire; but if the other options aren't possible, it will give you a sense of accomplishment and the education you need to move forward in life.

Graduation Ceremony No matter what source of education you use, you still have the privilege through tax payer money to participate in the graduation ceremony with your classmates. All you have to do is complete the graduation requirements and provide the proof to your school along with your request as early as possible. If the school does not satisfy your request; make them aware you know your rights and that you will alert the local newspapers, news stations, radio stations, public officials, rally up student support both through one on one contact and social networking sites, and any other resources you can think of. The idea is to put a little pressure on them so they know you mean business and will not back down! Trust me, they'll get the point and you'll get what you want!

College decisions may be difficult but if it's important to you, consider it seriously. Even if you struggled in high school, it doesn't mean you won't do well in college. Don't allow epilepsy to hold you back from studying and/or training for the occupation you desire. While you may not be able to be an airplane pilot, a police officer or join the armed forces or other jobs that could be potentially dangerous for you and/or your coworkers, you will be able to achieve most of the goals you set your mind to.

Today, there are people with epilepsy who are actors, authors, doctors, lawyers, scientists, teachers, sports professionals, musicians and, politicians, etc. See: *Famous People with Epilepsy*. There are very few barriers to keep you from achieving your future dreams. Your attitude might be the only wall preventing you from successfully moving forward.

Employment is certainly encouraged however you should be careful in choosing your work environment. You should always avoid working in places which would expose you to dangerous circumstances such as heavy machinery in factories or deep fryers in fast food restaurants, just to name a few.

If there's a possibility you could have a seizure at work, it is considerate to inform your boss *after* you have been hired. It's to your benefit for you to wait until you are hired in order to prevent hidden discrimination. Take note, it's against the law for an employer to fire you due to a disability. You are protected by the Americans with Disabilities Act.

Marriage and children is something most teenagers hope to experience, especially girls! Yes, you can get married and have healthy children! See: *Women and Epilepsy*

A Relationship with Your Parents

Being a teen with epilepsy is not only challenging for you but also for your parents. Ever since you came into their world as their little bundle of joy, they worried about your well being as most parents do. They shared their deepest concerns about keeping you safe. However, since you have epilepsy, they probably desire to protect you even more. If they are protecting you against your capabilities, you need to delicately help them recognize they're doing so. They need to know if they're not allowing you to expand into a mature teenager and eventually an independent adult. This doesn't mean you can twist and turn the situation to avoid discipline!

It may be hard for them to let you make decisions regarding your own activities, especially now that you're older. However with your help, school counselors, and the Epilepsy Foundation, they will be able to break free from their fears and help you glide your way into adulthood. Be the loving child they desire and yearn to protect. And take part in helping them help you in the transition. It's important that you work on it together. Encourage you parents to read, *Parenting Your Child with Epilepsy*.

True Stories

There are many things in life that have the potential to hold a person back from meeting their goals. For me being diagnosed with epilepsy at seven years old changed my life forever. As a young boy, I didn't quite understand the situation I was in or the challenges I would face as I grew up. Overcoming the challenges of intractable epilepsy and the limits of this disorder has been a major goal in my life so far.

Some of the major struggles I have faced have been the loss of my dream to play football, difficulties with my studies due to uncontrolled seizures, and facing brain surgery. I was instructed to no longer participate in contact sports between my sophomore and junior years of high school. That summer I spent time coming up with a new plan to keep myself active.

My plan was implemented when I joined the school's athletic trainer to help out with the sports programs in which I could no longer participate. As well as athletic training, I was able to focus more efforts on clubs and organizations in the school. I was elected into the National Honor Society, joined the Key Club, and became president of the Model Congress Club! During this time I was also able to increase my focus in Boy Scouts. I have achieved the rank of Eagle Scout and held the leadership role of Senior Patrol Leader for two consecutive terms!

Unfortunately, I continued to suffer from seizures. My grades began to slip due to memory loss and absences from school. This was one of my toughest times. I had to focus one hundred percent on my school work to try to keep my grade point average at the honor's level. Even with these obstacles, I was able to pull through some of my most difficult classes.

As time went on, my family planned for brain surgery, choosing this option with a 70% success rate to being seizure free! The surgical evaluation process took six months and included 32 inpatient hospital days causing weeks of missed school time in my junior year. Challenges grew as I struggled to keep my grades and activities at the high level I desired. I had my last seizure two days prior to surgery in November, 2006 for a left temporal lobectomy and partial removal of my hippo campus.

After the surgery, I went through a long and tiresome recovery and I needed to catch up on three weeks of school work. In the end, it is fair to say that epilepsy held me back from many things I wanted to do. More importantly however, it also helped me go in other rewarding directions with my life that I may not have pursued otherwise.

I also learned how to work harder in the face of obstacles, and now understand that success in life is not handed to you on a platter. Throughout life one must work for what they feel they truly deserve. I am now going on ten months seizure free!
K. Manning, Burlington Township NJ

I had epilepsy since I was ten years old. As a teen, I only had a seizure like every two or three years. I never told anyone about it. Only my close friends knew. College was a different story. I was fine until the second semester in college. I remember being in the cafeteria, chewing on a straw! Then all of a sudden, I woke up to my friends who I never told because it was still a new year. I didn't want any of them to know. They said they freaked out because they didn't know what to do. Luckily some kid, who was working there, knew what was happening.

So of course, I wasn't able to drive places, when I went home for breaks and such. Then it happened again in my sophomore year. Luckily I was in my room. One of my roommates was my friend from last year. She knew what was going on. Then it happened again in the spring.

When I went home once again, I couldn't drive. The year I moved into my apartment, my roommate already knew what happens. It kept happening for a while. I always felt so guilty because my friends had to pick me up and drive me everywhere. I felt like a burden. They said they didn't care. Even if they did, they didn't let me know. It was hard but I learned who my *real friends* were. They always looked out for me. When I would have a seizure, of course I'd get depressed for a while. I'd do the "why me" stuff. My friends were really good about it. I could really talk to them about it. They would make me feel better. I guess I let the stress get to me really bad those three years.
K. Taylor, Canton MI

As a teen, I had a hard time seeing my friends get their drivers license and going off with their girlfriends. I was just falling to the side and watching my friends live a "normal" life. I began to think to myself, "No girl would ever want to date a guy with epilepsy, who can't drive." So I didn't date or try to talk to girls. I would go to the store or where ever just watching the sidewalk under my feet as I walked.

Then one year when I was about sixteen, a new girl, Lisa moved into the neighborhood. I had such an awful crush on her. But with the frame of mind I was in, I would only say hello to her and keep walking. Lisa was sitting on her front porch, she said hello to me as I was walking. I don't know what made me do it but I went across the street over to where she was sitting and said, "Hello!"

She asked me why I always looked so depressed, like someone ran over my dog! I just told her, "I have epilepsy. I can't drive. Who would want to date a guy like me? No one would!" She looked me dead in the eyes and said, "I would!"

So we sat on her front porch swing for hours talking. She told me that she tried talking to me but I wasn't interested. I learned an important lesson that day. There are people who will accept you for who you are and all your flaws. There are people willing to look beyond and love you unconditionally. We dated for three years!
R. Hicks, Warren MI

I would have graduated with my class this year. But I had to drop out of school in ninth grade. That was very hard. I don't really have a lot of friends anymore because I haven't been in school for so long.

I studied at home to get my G.E.D. I struggled a lot on the test. I went back a few times to retest. I really could not focus. One day the lights really bothered me. I had just started a new medication, and I kept having problems with drowsiness during the test.

It is also very hard being a teen with epilepsy, watching people you know who are your age, getting their drivers license. I wanted to be just like them, graduating and driving. But I had to deal with staying home, and having my parents drive me everywhere. I couldn't get a job because I couldn't drive. It was too far to ask my parents to give me a ride every day.

I have been babysitting the kids around town since I was 12 years old. It was nice but I wanted to be like everyone else. I hoped that one day I could be on my own and drive to work. But there are some advantages for being home all the time. I wasn't around the drama in high school! I think that helped me mature a lot faster than other kids my age. I knew I would appreciate getting a car a lot more than I would have when I was younger. And I wouldn't take advantage of getting a job, like I would have when I was younger when things were given to me.

I knew that on the day I would get my license, and when I would get a job on my own, it would be the greatest accomplishment of my life! Only because I have been waiting for it for a long time (it seems like forever)! Anyway, last week, I finally got my G.E.D! My family is so proud of me because I did it all by myself! I worked through all the obstacles and did it! I "graduated" the same year as my class, just a few months later. But that was my goal and I did it! I feel like I am finally getting somewhere!
E. Alina, New Gretna NJ

I was in eighth grade in gym class when I had my first seizure. I was doing the stretches I did every day. The last thing I remember after stretching is waking up in an ambulance. I was scared. I didn't know where I was. I had to spend three days in the hospital. They wouldn't let me eat because they were afraid I would choke.

When my parents came to see me, they said the school's office said I admitted using and selling drugs by signing a paper! I remember the paper. My principal said I needed to sign it, so he would have proof that I sat in his office and discussed this with him. But that wasn't what the paper meant. It meant, I was pleading guilty to drug use, so I was expelled. There were no drug tests.

My neurologist said they have Neanderthal minds! It was all hearsay. They had no proof I was doing any drugs because I wasn't! They said that was enough to expel me so they did. From then on, the school gave me a lot of problems. There were a lot of classes that I wanted to take but they wouldn't let me without a slip from my doctor. I always had to sit out. I eventually went to school on line then they let me try "ehove" a vocational school.

I was in network, so I was able to visit all the classes, and stay in each one for a couple weeks. It's supposed to give women a chance to learn the stuff men do, such as electricity, welding, auto tech/body, diesel, etc. At the end of the year when it came time to pick a class for the next year, they wouldn't allow me to take any of them. They said it was too dangerous. I wondered why they let me come in the first place, if they weren't going to let me take anything! I had to go back to my home school that year and stayed a while. I had a seizure there, so I decided to go back to on line schooling again.

My school let my mom talk to the teachers about epilepsy, to educate them and show them how to aid a person who had seizures. The only questions they had were about liability. I don't even know if they listened. So far, I am still unable to get a license or a job.

My dad also has epilepsy. My neurologist is my dad's neurologist's son! We're supposed to be helping them because I guess they believe epilepsy may be hereditary, and they've been studying us. I'm not too sure. I barely talk to my doctors. They always talk to my mom. But they ask me how I'm feeling, etc.

The doctor thinks my hormones could have triggered some seizures, too. I had some bad periods so they put me on the birth control shot and it helped a lot! They gave me six months to be seizure free so I could get my driver's license. Unfortunately, I had a seizure last month and another one a couple days ago so I don't know if I'll ever able to drive.

People are nervous when I'm in there house because they think I'm going to have a seizure. But they just misunderstand. We know some people still believe you really can swallow your tongue! I was at my friend's house and had a seizure. Her dad put a plastic spoon in my mouth! Thank God it wasn't metal!

I don't feel all that abnormal since my dad has epilepsy, too. I don't mean I wish them on him. What I mean is I would feel worse if I were the only one. Our medication isn't cheap. My dad actually had to have a vagus nerve stimulator (VNS) implanted. I have grand mals and breakthrough seizures. They have done some damage. One time I blacked out for a second at the top of the staircase and fell down. It makes me scared and nervous when I can't control them. We just have to try to take care of ourselves, the best way we can and try to accept it.
B. Hensley, Sandusky OH

The first seizure I had (febrile) caused me to go into cardiac arrest. I didn't have any seizures again until seventh grade. I had a grand mal seizure in shop class. When I fell, I hit the corner of a grip vice right between my eyes. After an overnight stay in the hospital and a "million" tests later, my family doctor failed to follow up with me. I never grew out of the right-sided "tics." I twitched all the time, my head jerked to the side and my right arm contracted in weird ways. I couldn't control it.

When I moved to North Carolina to get a job as an EMS, I took my medical records with me. I looked at my old e.e.g. from eight years back. It read that I had an underlying seizure disorder! So I found a neurologist who ran more test. I didn't have another grand mal but I tend to have focal or tonic seizures with lack of sleep to this day.

I have a 3.5 mm brain damage to the frontal left lobe of my brain. I am a brilliant person in the medical field, I can remember everything! However, where the brain damage is located on my brain, my math level is that of a grade school child. If I didn't have this disorder, I would be in medical school! My primary care physician ignored my "tics," and twitches all throughout high school. He also ignored my e.e.g. results when I was 12 years old.

In high school, I was teased for my tics. My leg is turned at a 40 degree angle. Epilepsy caused so much right-sided weakness that I have a hip/leg defect. I have a 45 degree twist (rotation) in my tibia/fibia. I didn't think anything of it until now. I can hardly walk around the mall without having to stop and sit down. I'm going to have surgery to put a rod in my leg. It will keep my leg straight, and stay there for life, all because my physician ignored my signs, symptoms, and complaints.

I'm 25 years old now, and I didn't understand epilepsy until I took control over my own health care. Do I struggle? Sure! I hate taking the medication but I deal with it. I keep one mg. Ativan in my room because I can feel a seizure coming on within 20 – 40 minutes prior to the seizure. That is why I am allowed to drive and lead a "normal" life. I know I am not a freak. I do laugh about it only because you have to. But I do hate this. I count my lucky stars that I do have a drivers license, do not have grand mal seizures, and that I'm not a severe case. *S. Sekunda, Wilkes Barre PA*

I was eight years old when seizures hit me like a bat out of hell. No one knew why I was having seizures yet alone three types of seizures. The worst, of course was I had grand mals. My parents did everything they could. I saw a lot of neurologists, took more medicine that I thought was possible, and even had a right temporal lobectomy.

By the time I turned 11, my parents decided I should not live a protected life. So they checked with my doctor to see if I could go into softball. He said it was okay as long as I wore a helmet. So I started playing about a month later. My dad talked the coach about my "situation." She was really nice about it. He made sure she understood what to do if I had a seizure. And then my coach made my team mates learn seizure first aid. That was so cool. The best part was, none of them treated me differently. They actually seemed to look up to me. That's the first time I felt "free."

I made it through three practices without a seizure. But during the fourth, I had a grand mal. When I came out of it, everyone was really calm. They only seemed concerned about me. I learned later, that the coach handled it well, and my 12 year old team mate took care of me. I played the entire season but not without seizures.

The great thing was my coach insisted that the other teams in the league learned seizure first aid. My parents didn't think they would cooperate but the coaches were fully cooperative and supportive. I started the ketogenic diet that summer after the softball season was over. I've been seizure-free for six years, and medicine free for five years.

Katie, Williamsburg VA

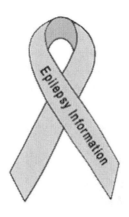

Success Stories
Plan to Succeed!

Confucius said, *"Our greatest glory is not, in never falling but in rising every time we fall!"*

Just because we're "dropped" physically from seizures doesn't mean we have to give up and give in. You can and probably already do have your own success story yet don't realize it. After reading this chapter, I hope you'll see you had or are living one you haven't recognized. No matter what, don't give up. Conquer your hardships with a passionate spirit and savor the victories of success whether big or small.

In order to grasp the intimacy of the following stories as well as to find your own, you need to know the definition of success. *Success* is the achievement of something desired, planned, and attempted. It doesn't say meeting your *maximum* desires and plans. Getting close to them can be a success story in itself. If you have a story that has reached even your least expectation you've succeeded! Keep this in mind. If you give up, and allow the wall of discouragement hold you back, you will stay there. *"Everything that has happened to you is either an opportunity to grow or an obstacle to keep you from growing. You choose."* Wayne Dyer.

Approach every day positively. See yourself rising above the condition that is trying to absorb your health. Think about the good in your life. Then think about the good that's possible in your future. That can be a struggle in itself but I assure you, you have a success story either now or coming your way. We all do. You have to stay positive. *"A pessimist sees the difficulty in every opportunity; an optimist sees the opportunity in ever difficulty."* Winston Churchill

First, I want to address a battle most of us have practiced. We have the temptation to wallow in self-pity. Do whatever it takes to stay away from it no matter how hard it gets. Your physical body may be weak but that doesn't mean your mind has to be. If you see yourself as strong, you'll be strong. Self-pity is a trap. *"What poison is to food, self-pity is to life"* Oliver C. Wilson

The true stories in this chapter show that people who also struggle with epilepsy have overcome negative feelings that epilepsy poses on all of us. Yes, we sometimes feel the need to hang our chins on our chest and give up but you need to fight that temptation! Instead, show the inner strength that you know is inside you.

Even though we may not all have super success stories, we all experience levels of success. Maybe it's getting a new medicine with fewer side effects. Or every period of time we enjoy being seizure free, maybe it's a year, a week or even a day. No matter what the length of time we spend living seizure free, it's considered successful because it's what we all desire. It may be temporary but it sure feels good! We need to consider each time we enjoy such precious moments, a success! It should "taste" as sweet as your favorite dessert!

Part of my success story does not include living a seizure free life. My success story is living with a lot less seizures. Having a success story and being happy doesn't mean everything is perfect. It means you've decided to set your mind to accept life as it is, see beyond the imperfections, and enjoy every sweet moment that's above the unfortunate norm.

In a unique way, we have something more special than the perfectly healthy people who are running around aimlessly through life. When we have that brief moment of success, we appreciate so much more than the people who don't have health problems. Personally, I think in a different kind of way, they're losing in life. Unless they've been through a personal tragedy they may never truly know how precious life is. We experience the taste of life that couldn't be more delicious when we enjoy a period of seizure free living.

I believe in the deepest depth of my soul most people who live completely healthy lives other than people who've experienced other forms of trauma, do not live life to the max nor appreciate it for what it's worth. They can't possibly know how precious life really is. I'll always see it that way. It's my hope that you will, too.

Our struggles have a unique way of helping us appreciate life even though our health is far from desirable. We need something that picks us up, and keeps us from feeling lost, hopeless, and helpless. I believe it's that brief moment of living seizure free. I enjoy every minute of every day that's seizure free. That's my true joy and success story. A joy I never knew before epilepsy touched my life. I hope you can find a way to enjoy those special moments as well, whatever they may be.

Everyone with epilepsy including me, can say without reservation that we've struggled with depression, feeling defeated, discouraged, alone, unloved, misunderstood, etc. However, I have stories to share with you that will help you see things in a different light. While reading the following stories, delete the emotions you feel as being a victim of epilepsy. Instead envision yourself as someone with the potential for your own success story regardless of your health. The more you fight to rise above it, the less it'll consume you. Yes it's difficult and disturbs a "normal" way of life but it doesn't have to be the center of your universe. You may have to deal with a lot of struggles but you can still experience and enjoy those sweet successful moments!

Never forget, your success story could be as simple as finally finding the perfect mix of medications to control your seizure activity *bet-*

ter. Even though that may be minor in your eyes, *better* is still a success and worthy of recognition!

Now you know success doesn't have to mean being seizure free or that you have to have a big exciting story. The following stories were collected long ago from my "friends" at Myspace. The following stories might not be yours or even close but they are encouraging, and may even be your *future* success story. Your story may even be better! That's a possibility that you should always look forward to.

True Stories

I don't know what it's like to live life without seizures. I started to have seizures when I was a baby. I get aggravated with people who complain about stupid things like their hair, their clothes, and even more stupid, their life! School has always been a battle for me. I get teased for days and even weeks after a grand mal seizure. It would be easy to sit down and cry, and worse give up. But instead I feel sorry for them. They don't understand what it's like to have the kind of battles I have. The sad part about that is, I can rise above it but I don't think they could. They're too busy focusing on other people, and trying to drag them down. I can't be dragged down. My parents would ground me!

All the trivial things I hear people whine about are just that, trivial. It makes me wonder what the heck they'd do if they had one seizure. Just one seizure! They'd be worse off than a sunken boat. But I can handle it because I learned that life doesn't revolve around me, and certainly not my health. My parents have always taught me that I am not the problem in my life. The seizures aren't either. They cause problems but they're not the problem. They're my strength.

My success story has nothing to do with living seizure free. I never have so I guess I don't know what I'm "missing." But what I do have is self confidence, strong will, and great parents. That's my success story.
Kayla, Reading PA

My story starts out as a very frustrated teenager. I started having seizures when I was 14. Now as an adult, I'm just beginning to understand all that encompasses my seizure disorder and the way it affects my life. After years of trying all kinds of medications and doses, and dealing with side effects, breakthrough seizures, and plain frustration in not being able to figure out that right balance, I got lucky. I, along with my neurologist finally figured out the right combination of medications and daily routine (sleep, eating habits, medication, stress, etc.) that worked. I was seizure free for three years.

Shortly after that three year mark, I started having seizures again, which has been attributed to me developing a tolerance to the medications. I went through another long period of time, when I was having seizures and feeling like I had no control over them. At one point in time, I was having tonic-clonic seizures (even though the typical seizures were complex partials). One day I had several tonic-clonic in the same day. A couple weeks later I think I had five in one day. It did get better in time, with medication management and watching my stress level. Trust me, it wasn't easy.

Two years later, I got pregnant. I had a few seizures (just partials) during my pregnancy and then none! Even with my medications, my baby is perfect. She is just about to celebrate her first birthday! I have now been seizure free for over 16 months! I feel the need to advocate the use of folic acid during pregnancy for women taking antiepileptic drugs. The risk for birth defects from your medications is cut in half by adding the recommended dose of folic acid to your daily medication regimen.

I guess the most important thing that I'd want to share with people is that it does no good to dwell in the bad. We have the power to learn and grow as a person, and to share things we've learned from having seizures. We can help dispel some myths and fears that others have about seizures and epilepsy. Yes, epilepsy is difficult. Yes, having seizures is scary and frustrating. Yes, it can seem as though there is no end in sight. But, no, it does not have to ruin your life. It does not

define you. It can only make you a stronger person. Perseverance is great fuel for self-confidence.
K. Eastin, St. Cloud MN

I started to have seizures when I was in sixth grade. I can remember like it was yesterday! I was in my physical education class when we had to square dance. Everything was fine except during the routines. I would stop and get "lost" for a few moments. I never suspected anything unusual until the following year. It continued while I was in mid-conversation with friends. It was very strange.

I had no idea what was happening until my first grand mal occurred. I was in advanced classes and I am sure sleep deprivation played a role at the time. My parents took me to three neurologists and finally settled with one that we all felt comfortable with. No one in my family has a history of seizures. This was my first one so the doctor did not diagnose me with epilepsy. However, the following week I had another grand mal at school. I was not happy! I did not understand what was happening to me or for what reason. I was prescribed an AED.

I do not remember very much of my seventh grade year besides not wanting to go to school and sleeping a lot! I continued to have seizures. My eighth grade year I was put on a different AED, and I ate everything in sight! Ha ha! I gained fifty pounds but the seizures did stop for a whole year. My neurologist was so impressed she pulled me off all my medication that summer. However when high school started in the Fall I had another grand mal the first week. I was so disappointed. Then I was switched to another AED, and I shed all of my weight in a matter of months! I could not believe it!

I was happy to be losing weight but I hated the attention I was getting. My high school life was pretty normal. In my freshman year, I skipped class with friends so often that I had to go to court! My parents were more disappointed than mad, which always made me feel worse because I was their "golden child."

I was still in advanced classes but my grades were terrible. I still never wanted to go to school. It was hard especially after I had a seizure. I really tried not to let it bother me though. I just went about my business like nothing had happened. All that mattered was my group of friends and me at the time. One thing in particular I remember was my sophomore year, when one of my best friends got a new car. I was so happy for her but I knew it would be a while before I would drive.

I remember having to get a state identification card because I was old enough to get into rated "R" movies but I did not have identification card! I still have it to this day! Ha ha! It seemed like high school would never end. However, I continued to shed pound after pound.

After another breakthrough seizure on the AED, I finally switched to another medication and another neurologist. The medical center in Houston seemed like the best place to find a solution. A pediatric neurologist at a children's hospital diagnosed me with generalized epilepsy and prescribed another AED. I remained seizure free for three years! During that time my weight stayed stable. Everything was fine. I just slept a lot as usual. I was not very thankful at the time but now that I look back, I am very thankful for the time I had! I accomplished more than most.

I can still remember the day I took my driving test when I was eighteen. I was so nervous I did not care about passing! I was just praying for it to end! Now that I look back at how angry I was at the world because I could not drive at the time, I am reminded that things happen for a reason. Several friends of mine had wrecked their vehicles at young ages. At least I can say I have respect for the road and respect for my vehicle.

I was so happy! I finally felt free and independent. I remember when I got my first speeding ticket! I was taking my friend home, and I had no idea I was speeding! When the cop pulled me over, my friend said "tell him to turn the lights off on his car that you have seizures!"

I said, "I don't think that's going to get me out of this one!" I finally felt free but that did not stop my mother from calling me all of the time! I suppose I would react the same way if my child was on the road and had epilepsy. I constantly tried to reassure her I would be okay. Sometimes you just have to have faith. Before I got my car, I would drive my parents' vehicles to school. Senior year had finally arrived. I even had a part time job! I transferred into regular classes and began to relax.

I really focused on my grades and looked towards the future. I had decided I wanted to pursue a career in nursing. The only thing holding me back from graduating was Spanish and my attendance record was still not great. I had to make up a few days before graduation but it worked out because I studied for Spanish constantly.

I was so nervous the week of finals. I went to every teacher to check my grades before graduation. I saved Spanish for last. Ha ha! I remember my teacher saying, "Ms. Jewell, I don't even know what you are worried about." I could have cried. Ha ha! No more Spanish for me! I graduated that week. One goal accomplished several more to go!
A. Jewell, Santa Fe TX

My story starts out as a very frustrated teenager. I started having seizures when I was 14. Now as an adult, I'm just beginning to understand all that encompasses my seizure disorder and the way it affects my life. After years of trying all kinds of medications and doses, and dealing with side effects, breakthrough seizures, and plain frustration in not being able to figure out that right balance, I got lucky. I, along with my neurologist finally figured out the right combination of medications and daily routine (sleep, eating habits, medication, stress, etc.) that worked. I was seizure free for three years.

Shortly after that three year mark, I started having seizures again, which has been attributed to me developing a tolerance to the medications. I went through another long period of time, when I was having seizures and feeling like I had no control over them. At one point in time, I was having tonic-clonic seizures (even though the typical seizures were complex partials). One day I had several tonic-clonic in the same day. A couple weeks later I think I had five in one day. It did get better in time, with medication management and watching my stress level. Trust me, it wasn't easy.

Two years later, I got pregnant. I had a few seizures (just partials) during my pregnancy and then none! Even with my medications, my baby is perfect. She is just about to celebrate her first birthday! I have now been seizure free for over 16 months! I feel the need to advocate the use of folic acid during pregnancy for women taking antiepileptic drugs. The risk for birth defects from your medications is cut in half by adding the recommended dose of folic acid to your daily medication regimen.

I guess the most important thing that I'd want to share with people is that it does no good to dwell in the bad. We have the power to learn and grow as a person, and to share things we've learned from having seizures. We can help dispel some myths and fears that others have about seizures and epilepsy. Yes, epilepsy is difficult. Yes, having seizures is scary and frustrating. Yes, it can seem as though there is no end in sight. But, no, it does not have to ruin your life. It does not define you. It can only make you a stronger person. Perseverance is great fuel for self-confidence.
K. Eastin, St. Cloud MN

What the heck, so what if you had a bad day! Tomorrow will be better! Go to bed and forget about it! When you wake up its a new day, another day you could either sit there and dwell how rotten yesterday was, or just get out of bed and hope today will be better I try to educate people about epilepsy through the use of humor. I personally would rather hear a good joke than sit through a lecture.

I was born with epilepsy so yeah I can make fun of myself since I am 39 years old. People have to learn to laugh at themselves and laugh with each other, not laugh at each other. I take medication to control my epilepsy. Too bad they don't make medication for stupidity! I know some people who would really benefit from it, if there was!

It is a bittersweet victory for me, because I have gone six months, and yet I think of those of us who haven't even gone one week which does sadden me. But I am happy for myself because it is a personal victory. I can honestly say this is the first summer I have enjoyed without a seizure. Not even as a little boy or even last year. I enjoyed this summer as much as I could. I wouldn't stay home! I would go to the park by the water fountain that kids play in. I even got in the fountain to cool off and kids would laugh at me! But I wasn't the only adult so I don't feel like a nut case! I have not missed one day of it. After work, I go there at night and watch the choreographed fountain light up to the music and think to myself, "It's amazing!" I think I enjoyed it more than I would have any other summer.

R. Hicks, Warren MI

I started having seizures when I was 11 years old. I was having grand mal seizures about once every three months. I would just fall and shake without any warning. At the time it wasn't that big a deal. Yeah it was confusing and the amount of injuries I had was continuous but it was livable.

When I was 17, I went straight into training to be a nurse. I was having a great time, yet over the next two years everything started to change. It increased to a seizure once a month, then once a week. It got to the point when it was every other day.

Understandably I was kicked out of nursing, lost a lot of friends because I was now their patient. I became nearly housebound. I was 19 years old. I had just moved into my own place, and it was tough. I had two or three friends who stuck around but the rest went off to live different lives, a life that I could never live. But I would never hold that against them. Not now anyway.

Five years later on really bad days, I was having up to three grand mal seizures and over 20 Petite mals a day. The only time I ever left the house in those five years was on Sunday's because it was my "assigned" day to be taken out by relatives. So I would plan all week on what I was going to wear, and how I was going to do my hair! I loved Sunday's and still do!

I was seven days away from my 25th birthday when I got a phone call from my specialist saying they wanted to see me immediately. What a pain in the butt that was because it wasn't a Sunday, and I didn't have a lift! When I got there and was told they had decided to operate, my exact words were "operate on what!?"

Eight a. m. the next day, they came for me and I was prepped for surgery. I had 17 operations on my right hand because I have Poland's Syndrome. I was used to hospitals and surgery but this one was different. I was scared as they were actually going to remove some of my brain!

My dad is my hero! He was the first thing I saw when I woke up. He was sitting by my bed crying. It's devastating to see your dad cry! I thought I was dead and that's why he was crying! I wanted to shout to him that it was okay but I couldn't move. I tried so hard but during the operation I had a stroke. It took over a year to learn how to walk and talk properly, and six months to learn how to read and write again.

A year later the good news was I had been seizure free for 384 days! I had moved back into my own house! I was in a new relationship, and started a new job! Everything was fantastic but while watching a firework display it started again. But it was different this time. I wasn't passing out and shaking anymore. Instead, I was having like an "abnormal consciousness," memory loss, hallucinations, visual, hearing, touch, smells, déjà vu & Jamais Vu, and nausea.

I was diagnosed with Temporal Lobe Epilepsy resulting in partial seizures and complex partial seizures. I had too much brain damage to be able to fix it and I had a probable hypothalmic hematoma (brain tumor on my hypothalamus). I was told to take the drugs and hope for the best. That was nine years ago. It took at least four years to get back to my old self again.

The trick was to surround myself with people who needed my help. I needed to feel useful again, to feel like I could mean something to someone, to not feel written off. I have about 15 - 20 seizures a day now. Sometimes you wouldn't notice but there are times when this condition is impossible to disguise. That's when the fight within you begins. You see it's not just about knowing facts with epilepsy or any disability it's about a little understanding and staying strong!
N. Peacock Newcastle, Upon Tyne, United Kingdom

I had been in love with alcohol since I was 17 years old. I would party all the time in high school and college. I would literally use alcohol to solve my problems. I don't want to say I was becoming an alcoholic but if I would have kept going, I probably would be. In November of 2006 I had a party at my house while my parents were gone. A few friends slept over and I was up all night.

The guy I was kind of dating at the time, left early in the morning. I got up, walked him to the door, and turned around to fall down and have a seizure. Luckily my best friend was there and she called 9-1-1. Prior to this, my other doctors just thought that it was lack of sleep that caused the seizures.

I had been taken to the hospital and underwent a series of tests. They made me come back a few weeks later to do a three day e.e.g. That is when they discovered that I had epilepsy. I started undergoing treatment. After a couple months of my doctor not seeing me and making me sit with the nurse, and telling me things like, "Everyone who has déjà is actually epileptic." I decided she wasn't the doctor for me.

I met my boyfriend in January of 2006. He had a traumatic brain injury after a car accident and so he went to an epileptologist. She has been treating me ever since and through a series of trial and error we discovered that some medicines would still causes me to have seizures. I've been on one a certain medication for about 16 months now and have been seizure free since!

I don't drink anymore unless it's an occasional wine cooler at a wedding or holiday party. I think finding out I was epileptic saved my life and my liver. I still have problems because dealing with epilepsy is hard, and I have it pretty good compared to some people. I have to limit what I eat, when I go to bed, what I drink, etc. Limiting yourself is very hard to deal with but I know that everyone with epilepsy is strong and that day to day we are all becoming stronger.
K. Murdoch, Howell NJ

I have three types of epilepsy, and for the first four to five years of being diagnosed, I was misdiagnosed with other types. I was doing well, until I saw the third specialist while in an inpatient treatment program. When I started puberty, my life changed, and continued to change because the seizures increased, like one wouldn't believe. Going from completely controlled to having major seizures every week, and having smaller ones throughout the whole time. I have been diagnosed with status epilepticus.

When the change came into my life more A.E.D.s were tried, joined together, so on and so forth. Three years ago, I found a new doctor, and in our very first meeting, she asked how I felt about the VNS, and if I knew anything about it. I had previously been turned down for 8 ½ years.

So having a doctor bring it up to me was amazing! I jumped on it! At that point I was taking 217 A.E.D pills a WEEK! And the seizures were nowhere near to under control. For most people, one or two types of A.E.D. will work, but not for me. I tried everything under the sun. Brain surgery was out of the question and most doctors said no to the VNS.

But my new doctor sent me to a big city hospital to have it done. They refused right before I was to be admitted into the program. My doctor called me and had me cancel all my appointments. The other doctors had already made their decision. She got the city of XXXXX certified to implant the VNS, and I was implanted! Yes, I was the first! It has been a God send! I am completely off A.E.D.s, and worked full time for two and a half years!

I am now returning to college full time! My life has done a complete 180 degree turn around from three and a half years ago. I was implanted in July 2004. My implant was turned on August 2004. I only take vitamins to keep my body healthy. If I don't, and get any kind of infection or anything, I will start having seizures.
R. Endres, Brainerd MN

After a switch in medication when I was younger (I forget when exactly the switch was) the seizures were under control. The seizures happened between fifth & eighth grade. When I was 18, I started driving, being seizure free for more than the required time to drive.

I probably would have been able to drive at 16, but the lack of money for a car was more of an issue than the seizures at that point. So, just in the way a change in medicine worked for me and allowed me to drive in the end is my story.
Carol

I'm writing a blog in hopes I can meet someone with a seizure disorder like mine, so my friends and family have a better understanding. I started having seizures when I was 13. At that time I had no idea what they were. I never told anyone because I didn't really think anything of it. My world didn't come crashing down until I was fifteen. I was in math class taking a final, and started having strange blackouts one after another. I kept forgetting where I was and what I was doing. I went to the nurse and got sent home.

When I got home I had, what we later found out was, a grand mal seizure (generalized tonic-clonic). After having a grand mal you can't remember anything, you're dazed, sore, and tired. My mother told me that I complained of a headache, then my eyes rolled back and my body starting convulsing. She said blood and bubbles were coming out of my mouth. She thought I was dying. It's scary, but it's reality. My first doctor misdiagnosed me. He put me on enough medication for a 300 pound man! The meds made me depressed, suicidal. I became a person I could no longer recognize.

I gained so much weight due to the overdosing caused by my crazy doctor. It's like I wasn't living anymore. I found a new doctor, and told him how all the seizures happened during my period. He said the seizures were caused by low estrogen levels which happen during that time of the month. Granted I still have some petit mals when not menstruating but, petit mals aren't that bad. They last as long as a blink, and I forget what I was doing or saying. Grand mals can last five minutes and can cause damage.

I do worry that one day a seizure will cause brain damage or turn me in to a vegetable. But it no longer controls my life. I can sense when I'm going to have them now. I finally felt like the real me. My doctor tried stopping my period with birth control. However when you're on meds, your liver works harder. So the birth control didn't work. My liver was killing it before it could. My doctor won't let me try birth control alone. I'm hoping I will find a doctor who will let me go on birth control alone. Stopping my periods can stop the seizures. Until then I'll just have to deal with them.
L. Oliver, Mt. Pleasant PA

I was undiagnosed until I was almost 18, but I had seizures as long as I can remember. Even so, I still graduated from high school. I was diagnosed when I was taking an extra year of building and construction classes, and a class "A" truck driving, so I never got my truck driving license. I have always held a full time job. The job I have now I've had for ten years. I started at when I was 19 years old. I was lower management for two years, but that's when the seizures were the worst.

I got married at 21 years old and built our house the following year. A couple years later my wife and I, had a healthy baby girl! We've decided that Riley is healthy, and one is a good number. Besides, we both work in social services.

After meeting my epileptologist for the first time, she asked me for as close of a description of my life history as I could give. Including what doctors I had seen, and what meds I had taken etc. And then she promptly congratulated me for not only surviving this long, but carrying on a productive life style! When as a teen it would have been so easy to give up and achieve nothing.

I work full time, am married, and have a child. I have made a few alterations to accommodate my epilepsy, but I'm making the best of it. My point is that for anyone younger who is diagnosed, it can feel like the end of the world, but I got all the things I wanted done before I turned 30. My life is altered a bit to fit my needs, but with any luck that will change soon, too. I wish I had been a little less hesitant to have the surgery ten years ago. Three months after my partial lobectomy was done, I am still seizure free. I'm working full time, and looking forward to getting my driver's license back. I had my VNS turned down once, and have started reducing my Lyrica.

I'm looking forward to taking my computer aid drafting class, again. I had stopped because my ability to concentrate and retain anything I read was gone. I'm hoping that it gets better now. I'm still grasping the fact that I am seizure free!
B. Webster, Gray ME

My first seizure was when I was 25 years old at work stocking shelves and woke up to a bunch of "uniforms." They already had an IV in my arm. Apparently I had a bad enough seizure that I scared some new guy from coming back to work.

At that time, I had no clue what was going on. I had two little kids and a wife. I knew whatever was happening was bad and bigger than me. After a month of seizures, about five a week, all I could think about was how am I going to feed my family and pay the bills? What if my wife leaves me? Will my kids be afraid of me?

I have no clue why I had that first seizure or even why I have them at all. But I was diagnosed with epilepsy six months later. My life was spinning out of control. I had seizures in front of my wife and kids. That always brought the worst out of me. I searched for a doctor that knew what they were doing. My new doctor, after putting up with five jerks, is awesome. He helped get the seizures controlled a lot better and my attitude, too. I was bitter. He helped my wife learn how to put up with all my crap and all the other things she had to deal with. I still have seizures. I take a lot of medicine but the seizures aren't near as often.

But I feel like I beat the battle over epilepsy. I have a steady job, I go to the gym with some friends, and I have a family who stands behind me. They treat me good. My wife stayed by my side from the very beginning. She deserves a medal. I was an angry person. My life changed, but it's different now and in a lot of ways it's better. I know I'm closer to my kids than I ever would have been. And I love my wife more than I ever could have imagined.

My success story has nothing to do with getting seizures out of my life. It's becoming a better person than I know I would have been. I don't know what my wife saw in me. But I'm glad she sees something in me now, and it's not the epilepsy. That's my success story. My name is William and I always went by Bill until my wife started calling me Will. She says it because I have the will to live a normal life.
Will, Farmington NM

In the fall of 1989, I was coming home from a late lab (college class). It was dark and rainy, and I was tired. A deer jumped out in front of me. The last thing I remember was stomping the brake pedal & asking God to help me. The deer came up over the hood & through my windshield. I guess it must have struggled to get out, because it kicked me in the head. If you know anything about deer, you know their hooves are like razors. The next thing I remembered was being in the emergency room getting stitched up.

The seizures didn't start right away they started about a year after I had my first child in '94. They didn't start out as seizures they were more like "auras." My ears would ring everything looked like the TV when the cable is out. But worse of all, I got this funny metallic taste. The "auras" never lasted more than 10-20 seconds.

When I had the first seizure I was so terrified I went straight to the emergency room! When I described the symptoms, I was told I was having a panic attack and sent home! They were very sporadic, and since I didn't have them every day (or week, or even month) I went along with my life as usual. I kept working, and I even kept driving. It TERRIFIES me to know I could have hurt or killed somebody. I also had two more children.

Fast forward to 2002! My oldest son was in school, and his little brother & sister were home with me. I had a seizure *not an aura* in the kitchen. I distinctly remember coming out of it wondering where I was, and who these kids were. Something had to be wrong, so I scheduled an appointment with my family doctor. She referred me to a neurologist.

When I had an MRI, and actually had a seizure while I was in the machine. I was diagnosed with temporal lobe epilepsy. I don't con-vulse, I make a face as though I'm in pain, and I clench my fists, and chew. Sometimes I fall over, but not always. It can take as long as 30 minutes for me to "come back." I'm on Trileptal after trying Topamax, Carbatrol, Zonegran, and Lamictal. The Topamax worked the best for the seizures and migraines, but I had to stop taking it due to some serious side-effects. The pressure in my eyes was raised. The seizures are somewhat under control, they only seem to hit around my period

now, before during or after. I'm 41 year old mom of three kids. None of my children have any signs of epilepsy.
Karen, Eastern OH

Years ago, when I was in high school, I heard a boy talk about his success in the same paragraph as the fact he had epilepsy. At that time, I thought success and epilepsy were an oxymoron. I didn't believe life could be successful when you had epilepsy. I thought that boy was confused or simply bonkers! But now that I'm married with two children, I see what he was enjoying back then was a possibility.

Now, I have a life that many people who are completely healthy desire but don't have! My husband understands and has an amazing amount of patience when it comes to epilepsy, especially the lack of memory part. Not only is he patient and loving but he's taught my children to be the same way.

If I would have continued to allow epilepsy to make me feel less than other people or incapable of a normal life, I'd be alone and sad right now. But I'm thankful for my family and friends. They helped me realize I'm no less than anyone else in this world! They pushed me into thinking, believing, and knowing that I have a purpose in life and that it's important to find it.

I did find it, when I married my husband and had two children who are active in helping other people with disabilities. I never told them to do that. They just do it because of the way they see me. They want people with disabilities to enjoy feeling loved and accepted the way I am. Now I see myself as normal and I believe my life is successful. I'm thankful for the people in my life who lead me in that direction. To me, successfulness doesn't mean being famous or doing some overly fantastic thing it's about living life in a complete fashion just like the outside world does. I'm not less than anyone else, and I have a life that proves that.
Deborah, Burlington VT

When I think about success in my life, some people would think I'm crazy for calling them a success. Some people would just be happy for me but not recognize them as a success.

I remember when I was in college, and finished my first semester. It was a long hard semester and I only had two seizures! I was so excited about that. But no one seemed to understand my excitement. I'm sure some of my friends and family thought I was studying too hard! But they don't know what that felt like for me. I don't wish something like that on anyone but I wish they could know the difference between perfect and great. There is a difference. Perfect is nothing is wrong. Great is things do go wrong until they take a break. That's great to me. I don't know if anyone else would agree with me but that semester was a success story. I'm thankful for it.

The strange thing is I didn't even realize it until the semester was over and I had a breather. What's even stranger is that I was living my life in freedom and didn't realize it. That says to me that epilepsy doesn't make me happy or sad. It's just a distraction from the things I want to concentrate on.

D. Simmons, Ottawa, Canada

In the beginning of my battle with epilepsy, I fought (sometimes literally!) to be heard and believed that I was truly having seizures. I was having grand mal seizures at night and atonic during the day which was obviously above all the neurologists education with whom I desperately sought help. It was hard to hang in because it felt like it would take forever for a doctor to believe that I was having seizures yet alone help me. But I never gave up or quit believing that someday, I wouldn't have to fight to be heard, respected, and properly treated (medically).

As I waited, I clung to the precious verse of Joshua 1:9, *I command you, be strong and courageous! Do not be afraid or discouraged, for the Lord is with you wherever you go.* I don't know how I would have handled it emotionally without that promise because my greatest battle was discouragement. At times, I felt like it was never going to get better.

It's easy to get discouraged when the doctors who are supposed to help you, don't even believe you and won't help you. But that incredible moment finally came when my epileptologist said I was having seizures. As insane as it seems, I was thrilled to hear those words! I was finally vindicated! I was going to be respected again and finally get the help my brain needed. I felt whole again! I knew my life was going to turn around. I knew I was going to be able to look forward to every new day, again.

Diane

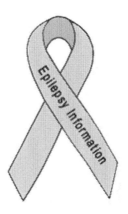

A Different Look at Epilepsy

It can be hard to find a way to explain what epilepsy and seizures are like to people who never experienced them. I tried to come up with definitions to cover both but that's absolutely impossible! Epilepsy and seizures are far too diversified from one person to the next. However, when you compare the analogies below, you can see some consistency. After all, we all have violence in our brains, and we all have very poor memory. I'm thrilled to share all the analogies presented to you by my "friends." from social networking sites. I hope they'll help you understand the way other "patients" view epilepsy and seizures. And maybe you'll have a little fun at the same time.

Seizure:

They're like a lightning storm that goes off in my brain.
J. Mooney, Dayton OH

They're like a pot of noodles that get over boiled. Then bubble up and spill all over.
Jessica, Kansas City MO

A seizure is like an earthquake! You lose your footing, everything collapses around you, you fall, and everyone panics!

K. A. Doyle, East Waterboro ME

It's like putting your brain on an electric fence!
R. Gerstner, Winter Haven FL

It's like a thunderstorm in your head with a flood of water flowing out of your mouth.
Katie, Las Vegas NV

For me, when people ask me, I tell them my brain is having its own little thunder storm. The messed up brain activity is the erratic lightening and the seizure is the thunder. As some of us know, there might be an occasional downpour! It lasts from anywhere from 30 seconds to two minutes.

I have a Huge headache and sleep for a long time afterward. I never know when it's going to storm again. But the next day, there will be sunshine! Of course, there's a lot of hand gesturing when I tell people!
D. Dinstett, Portage MI

Unfortunately, I'm coherent. I feel like I'm gasping for a breath then immediately after, exhaling with a forceful thrust while someone's performing the Heimlich maneuver all at the same time. It's so scary. I fear and feel like I'm going to die.
Diane

Seizures are like a storm or tornado going on inside my head. When you "wake up" it's like trying to put the pieces back together, and looking at the aftermath. My doctor says it's like an electric short. When the wire shorts out, the message doesn't get to the brain, and that's when the seizure happens. That helped me understand what the heck was going on inside my head. When everyone else was trying to explain it to me, I just didn't get it until the doc said what he did.
K. Binkley-Pelfrey, Waverly TN

Having a seizure is like when the power goes out and your computer shuts down, and is in safe mode. It doesn't come on and go right back to where you left, and has to reboot. *L. Oliver, Mount Pleasant PA*

Epilepsy:

The best way I can describe epilepsy is it's like you're a remote control toy that runs great until the batteries die (the batteries are the seizure of course.)
Jennifer, Springfield MA

It's like Dory (with a really bad memory) from the cartoon, Finding Nemo!
Y. Johnson, Denver CO

It's like being closed up in a trap. You look around and see how all the other kids are able to drive, play sports, go to dances, etc. They go where you can't go because you have to be watched and be cautious. Plus you don't know who your friends are and who aren't. *K. Fenstermaker, Cleveland OH*

Epilepsy is like a long and winding road. You never truly know what's around the bend, good or bad.

R. Newhall, Wichita KS

It's like an earthquake, unpredictable and a little scary but when the hard part is over, you realize how truly lucky you are!"
A. Faure, Valley Stream NY

Epilepsy's like an itch you can't scratch! Difficult to be comfortable and can't be ignored.
W. J. Hurren, Fort Worth TX

Having epilepsy is like living in the *Wizard of Oz* movie. Even though your friends are by your side, you never feel safe because you don't know when the witch (seizure) is going to jump out and get you.
Diane

It's like a flower bud that never gets sunlight or water. It's holding back a person who's ready to bloom into a full blown beautiful creation but is held back by outside influences such as seizures, medication, and self esteem. It's like something else has taken over the right side of my body.

When I have a grand mal seizure, I actually have a nightmare. My body feels like its melting. It's what I picture burning in hell would be like. So, I guess you could say epilepsy is like a "nightmare," in "hell", or...well, I can't think of a word to describe the part of taking over my hand!
B. Cunningham, Gastonia NC

Epilepsy is like living in a haunted house. You deal with a lot of fear wondering when the seizure will jump out and scare you. You never truly feel safe.
Kelsie, Bethesda MD

When you have epilepsy, a part of it is like having Alzheimer's because your memory barely functions.
Katie S.

It's like having A. D. D., dementia, paralysis, muteness, and a brief coma, all scrambled up into one person which causes complete disarray in your life. It's hard to concentrate on any one thing for a lengthy amount of time, especially when reading. It's also hard to remember things like what day, week, month, season, and even year. It gets frustrating because it makes me feel as if I'm dumb when I know I'm not.
Tori

It's Just the Way They See It!

Epilepsy is like a roller coaster ride, full of ups and downs and sudden turns! Even though the ups and downs and sudden turns sometimes get the best of us, we can take advantage of the ups and/or create some! Some of us tend to come up with a few silly comments in order to take the edge off a very serious moment. With that in mind, the following comments were made by my "friends" from a collection of social networking sites.

Epilepsy is definitely serious but humor helps when all else fails. It also helps other people feel a little more comfortable after witnessing a seizure. When we use humor they find it easier to relax and/or "recuperate" from their emotional trauma. Please note, I am not saying it's alright for other people to make fun of you, the seizures, or epilepsy. People in the "outside world" may not be doing it to take the edge off a very serious moment. They may be doing it to be mean and callous. But let's disregard them, and enjoy this chapter as friends with a lot in common.

Keep in mind that the following comments are for personal use. They are not promoted by me. I'm simply passing along what other people have shared. They found a way to take the moment of fear and concern away from the viewer(s) of a seizure or anyone who uncomfortably got their selves involved in a conversation about epilepsy. They managed to turn those uneasy moments into a different atmosphere using fun and/or humor. Epilepsy and seizures are still recognized as serious yet the humor is a part or maybe most of what they'll remember. It may give them a different idea of how you see yourself and how you want them to see you.

Remember that your reaction has the strongest expression of authority. You may not have control over seizures or epilepsy as a whole but you can have control over the end result. Your comment may be more memorable during that conversation and/or the seizure itself. The bottom line is, if you treat it differently, others will too.

Please don't get insulted or offended by any of the following comments. If you do, you're missing the purpose. Feel free to adopt any of the following phrases so you can help alleviate tension during those uncomfortable moments.

People ask me how I stay in such good shape. I tell them to check out my video . . . *"Twitching Along with Sherry!"*

Brain surgery left me with bumps on my skull from the hardware that put it back together. When I talk to people about my surgery, I try to get them to feel my skull. They usually reply by saying, "Eww, that's disgusting!" But I quickly reply, "It's not any different than the knuckles on your hand. I guess that makes me a genuine *knuckle head!*"

"I have a great memory, it's just short!"

I usually point and say to the person of choice, (usually whoever is closest), "It's your fault!"

I'm okay. This happens all the time when I think of my mother in law!

I think David (in the Bible) had it easy. He only had to deal with one Goliath!

My seven year old son tells people after he had a seizure that his brain flipped out and went crazy! Another one is that his brain just got done exercising!

My youngest son had a new type of seizure for his last four while standing up. My older son was standing close to him during the seizure to keep him from getting hurt. While my youngest son was having the seizure, he "peed" on him! So he's been going around telling everyone, "I "peed" on my brother, and I didn't even get in trouble!"

People who have seizures make the best break dancers!

After a seizure someone would say, 'You just had a seizure!' So I'd throw them off balance and say, "I didn't have a seizure, my brain did!"

My son told his classmate and friend, "Mom's brain just went on tilt. She'll be out of order for a little bit!"

When you have a seizure in front of your peers and they insist on teasing or insulting you, tell them you weren't having a seizure, you were practicing "stop, drop, and roll" so when you *visit* them in hell, you won't burn, too!

Some people's memory is shot! "I've got a great memory. What was your name again?"

The scarecrow wants to meet the Wizard of Oz so bad because he doesn't have a brain. Personally, I think he's lucky he doesn't have a brain!

Yes, I did just have a seizure, but I was only temporarily out of order!

I thought you knew I had brain surgery after all it's a no-brainer!

When I'm around people that know I had a lobectomy (at least a golf ball size of my brain removed,) and I can't come up with a word, I say, "You'd be that way too if you were an airhead!

When I have "little" seizures, my children say, "Mom's brain just went out to lunch she'll be back shortly!" Or if I grounded one of them, they will say, "Oh Mom you didn't ground me, you just had a little seizure." I just have to laugh at it sometimes! It makes life less serious and more fun!

I must have had too much soda. I got all shook up and foamed all over!

I don't understand why people today get all upset over seizures. I thought "rock and roll" was popular!

No one told me the weather was supposed to be bad today. I guess I'm the only one that got struck by lightning!"

Some people are troubled by this, others just laugh, and still others just nod and move on. We say, "Hey we can't drink, but we can be fun at parties. All we have to do is have a seizure. Then we'll throw a drink to be shaken, not stirred in our hands, and call ourselves bartenders!" I know that sounds bad to some but humor, dry or not helps!

I just got a job as Tickle Me Elmo. I was only practicing!

Terminology on a Personal Level

Words can make a significant difference in the world of epilepsy.

Since I've had the privilege of being the "epilepsy advocate" on many social websites, I had a lot of opportunities to dig into people's brains. Only I didn't make the money, brain surgeons do for digging into people's brains! Since I think the subject of terminology affects everyone who has epilepsy, I posted the following comment by my friend from the U.K. so that my friends could respond with their opinions.

Posting: At "Uni" today the lecturer was referring to a seizure as a fit. I know how many people prefer the word seizure. Personally for me when I think of fit, I think of a fit of laughter or anger. I don't think epilepsy. I'm going to email the speaker and ask her to change her terminology or people will never learn anything different. I feel it's very important for people who are teaching others to have the preferred terms. I just wondered how many people prefer the term seizure over fit.

They responded with the following comments...

I totally agree. "Fit" is completely inappropriate and a little insulting. If you're having a seizure just name it for what it is, a seizure!

They are seizures plain and simple. Seizure is the medical terminology and fit is just not acceptable. It sounds ignorant. A "fit" is a brat's way of getting what they want! A seizure is the brain's way of getting what it wants!

Our son Dallas has epilepsy and has seizures when the brain waves aren't working right. That is the difference between those two.

I prefer seizure!

Fit sounds ancient to me, and disturbs me a bit. I don't like the sound of it, let's call it what it is!

Fits are for kids! Unfortunately the lecturer probably heard a doctor use the word fit. They are the worst for not knowing the difference!

I refer to it as a seizure. How can someone say it's a fit when they're all different? I mean, when I had epilepsy and had a psycho motor seizure, I just stared. Is that a fit?

I prefer seizure over fit any day!

Fit is an out of date back woods term! Most people with epilepsy would find the term offensive. Fit sounds like someone having a tantrum and is belittling. It does not take a rocket scientist to know it is much kinder to refer to the seizure as what it is, a seizure!

Seizure is the term, the medical profession uses, and most with the sensitivity and an ounce of respect for anyone suffering from such a neurological disorder.

I prefer the term "seizure." But I also recognize that people in the UK refer to seizures as "fits." They aren't referring to the spoiled brat kind, either! People of my grandparent's generation always referred to seizures as "fits." It's just a figure of speech.

I would rather call it a seizure because when I have a fit, I'm usually yelling at someone or disagreeing.

Seizure!!!!!!!!!!!!!!!!!!!!!! Without a doubt!!!!!!!!!!!!!!!!!

Calling it a fit trivializes the enormity of the pain we go through. It is pretty much saying, "oh well, she had a fit." Calling it a seizure makes it real and puts it out there. Why should we pretend it's something it isn't?

People are able to control their anger or "fits." I wish I could have control over the seizures. A change is in order. Definitely seizure! "Fit" sounds demeaning.

What's with the deal that people think they can pick and choose what they call anything other than the medical name? I think they should be called idiots! After all that's what they are!

I prefer seizure. It makes me think of some brat who's belligerent because they are not getting their way!

Seizure, period!

It's starting to get annoying how politically correct we have to be these days. What happened to sticks and stones? People need to stop being offended by such silly things, and start focusing on what really matters.

I find even the fact that this question is being asked to be a bit of an insult.

Of course we should refer to seizures as what they are, seizures!

When I think of a fit, I think of a fit of laughter or anger. I don't think of epilepsy.

Personally I prefer the word seizure.

A fit is someone who is throwing a fit because they didn't get their way with something!

A fit is not a seizure! This person needs to rephrase her words when she is speaking about seizures.

I'm very against that word fit being used in that format. They kept telling me that my son, Dallas was just throwing fits, and I needed to get control of him. This was before they diagnosed him with seizures, when he was actually having seizures.

I prefer the term seizure. When I think of a fit, I think of a three year old child throwing a tantrum!

I completely agree the word that should be used is seizure. Typically, one says, "He threw a fit about it," as in someone is outraged at something or if a young child is having a temper tantrum. Involuntary seizures involve neither description.

I do believe calling an epileptic seizure a "fit" is a negative connotation. It must only be those who have this condition that know the difference. As well as for those who are friends and family of someone with epilepsy.

Having a "fit" does bring to mind a child throwing a tantrum or some-one in a "fit of rage."

There is so much in which people don't know about this condition. It does seem like there isn't much care going into finding information, except by those like us who have epilepsy.

Either I prefer seizure or spell but not a fit. Fits are what little children throw when they don't get their way! Yup, I should know. I was raised with nine brothers and sisters. Being the eldest they knew how to throw it then I threw it right back at them!

I prefer the term seizure because it's more technically accurate for the action. Also, the term fit could be perceived as derogatory by either the person having the seizure or the by-standers who witness it. The term "fit" describes a dress size or someone angry! So the best descriptive word for seizure is seizure!

When I was training to be a nurse, seizure was the medical term for grand mals (generalized tonic-clonic), and for people who didn't have a history of epilepsy. "Fit" i.e. "attack" was used for partial or complex partial seizures.

I've also noticed that Americans and American TV programs use the word seizure while as in the UK, fit and convulsions is used more than seizure. I don't think there is a right word for it. I think it's a personal thing.

I prefer seizure but my European and Aussie friends use the term "fit" quite a bit.

I prefer seizure. I agree with the tantrum comments.

I think people should call it what it is, a seizure! Cancer eats people alive but you don't see people calling cancer, the eating disease. I see no reason why seizures should be called fit or any other degrading word.

With all that said, let's see how the following books define both seizure and fit:

Second College Edition dictionary:

Seizure: A sudden paroxysm, as an epileptic convulsion

Fit: A sudden acute attack of a disease. A sudden appearance of a symptom such as coughing, convulsion, sudden outburst of emotion, fit of jealousy, sudden period of vigorous activity. With irregular intervals of action and inaction; intermittently hardship

Webster's thesaurus of the English language:

Seizure: convulsion, break down

Fit: attack

So the bottom line is it's a personal thing. I don't think it matters what the definitions are in both the Webster's dictionary and thesaurus. What really matters is the way the person using the word is intending it to mean, as well as the person hearing the word receives it. What offends you might not even catch another person's attention. Apparently, it boils down to you and your sensitivity, as well as personal desire for respect. If you prefer the word seizure over fit, be sure to let the people in your life know your preference with expectation they'll respect your choice of terminology.

Medical

Information

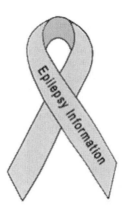

Tests

Doctors can say what he or she thinks but that isn't good enough! Seizures are serious business. Every seizure you experience, adversely affects you. You do not have the luxury of playing guessing games with your precious brain! Your doctor shouldn't either! If they have not performed any tests, you need to take charge of your health. Insist on well-rounded testing which will be the introduction to getting the medical care you deserve.

The purpose of initial testing is to not only prove or disprove seizure activity but also to determine the seizure frequency, duration, types, and clues of abnormalities. Even if you think, you know what types of seizures you are having and how often, you may be wrong! You could be having subtle seizures undetected by you. Once you have received all the necessary information, you can get started with the best treatment plan designed specifically for you.

Expect the following tests as you attempt to gain control over seizures:
- Blood work
- CT/CAT scan
- E.E.G.
- Medical history

- M.R.I.
- Neurological examination

Blood Tests

Increase the safety and efficacy of drug therapy in epilepsy.

Purpose:
- Determines how your body absorbs and eliminates each type of medicine.
- Checks medication levels, to ensure they are in the desired range for liver health.
- May tell the doctor whether you have been taking the medicine as prescribed.
- Find metabolic or genetic disorders that may be associated with seizures.
- Find underlying problems such as infections, lead poisoning, anemia, and diabetes that may be causing or triggering the seizures.
- See if the medication is within the desired therapeutic range.

D.E.X.A. *a.k.a.* D. X. A.
(bone densitometry)

Enhanced form of X-ray technology used to measure bone density. The following AEDs can cause calcium absorption interference followed by bone loss:
- Depakote
- Dilantin
- Tegretol (including XR)
- Carbatrol
- Phenobarbital

This list is not all inclusive. Investigate the medication you take and the effect on your bones. No matter what medication you take, a DEXA study is highly recommended.

Preparation:

- You may follow your regular daily routine.
- Take your medications as usual.
- At least 24 hours prior to the exam, do not take vitamins or calcium supplements.
- Avoid garments that have metal zippers, belts or buttons. (Sweat pants with an elastic waist band. Women are encouraged to wear a sports bra).
- Leave all jewelry at home.
- Do not wear body piercings.

Procedure:

- You will lie on a large padded table.
- An X-ray *generator* will be located beneath you.
- An arm-like imaging device is approximately 18" above your face.
- Your legs will be flat for the first part then laid on a padded box the second part.
- You must stay very still.
- The detector slowly passes over you.
- The test is very quiet, equivalent to a low hum.
- *The radiation is very low therefore, the technologist may sit right next to you!*
- *The test ranges from 5 – 10 minutes.*

After procedure:

- You may return to your normal activities.

Benefits:

- The procedure is painless and noninvasive.
- Small amount of radiation.
- Most accurate method available.
- Widely available.
- Performed on an outpatient basis (usually in hospitals).
- No radiation remains in your body.
- You may return to your regular routine immediately after the test.
- Advantages outweigh the risks.

Disadvantages:
- Limited use in people with a spinal deformity who had previous spinal surgery.
- Presence of vertebral compression fractures or osteoarthritis may interfere with the accuracy of the test.

Risks:
- There is always a slight chance of cancer from radiation. However, the benefit of an accurate diagnosis far outweighs the risk.
- The effective radiation from the procedure is about the same as the average person receives from the environmental radiation in one day. Therefore, the increased risk of cancer is comparable to the risk to what is acquired by living one more day!

It's very important to follow up with the DEXA test. The regularity depends on the result of the previous study or a change in your height. Calcium taken with vitamin D but separate from iron can fight bone conditions caused by a.e.d.s.

BRAIN SCANS

One of the most important ways in diagnosing and treating epilepsy is through brain scans. Everyone's brain is unique therefore, brain scans help doctors narrow in on the specifics necessary to perform their task of helping you regain control over seizure activity. Brain scans reveal changes, structural abnormalities, damage, and activity of the brain.

C.T. *a.k.a.* C.A.T.
(Computed Tomography)

Detects brain damage, and highlights local changes in cerebral blood flow (a measure of brain activity). The scanner works very much like an X-ray machine. To visualize the process, imagine looking at one end of a loaf of sliced bread. If you pull a slice out of the loaf, you can see the entire surface of that slice, from the outer crust to the center. Your brain can be seen on CT scan "slices" in a similar way, from the outside to the center. The exam produces multiple slices showing multiple views of the area being examined. The "slices" can be displayed on a video monitor and saved on film for analysis.

Preparation:
- Clear liquid breakfast (for tests scheduled in the morning).
- Clear liquid lunch (for tests scheduled in the afternoon).
- If you are claustrophobic or have chronic pain, you make take a mild sedative.

Procedure:
- The first part of the test will be without contrast.
- You will lie on a narrow table that slides into the circular opening of the scanner.
- An IV line will be started.
- Your head will be put in a "holder" with a strap across your forehead.
- The table will move slowly through a donut shaped scanner.
- You'll see temporary *lights,* which ensures the technician you're in the proper position.
- During the test, the machine sounds something like an airplane preparing to lift off and clicking sounds.
- You must stay still.
- The technologist will be able to see you through a leaded glass, as well as hear you and speak with you at all times. You will be able to respond using a microphone.
- The table will then move slowly through the scanner again during the test.
- You will hear a spinning-like sound during the test.
- Directly after part one of the test, an IV contrast is used.
- You'll feel a warm, flushed sensation from the contrast. You may even feel as though you are urinating!
- You may experience a metallic taste with a possible scent of alcohol (lasts 1 – 2 minutes).
- You may experience mild discomfort from stillness for several minutes.
- You will be alone inside the exam room during the scan.
- *The test is usually completed within 10 minutes.*

Pediatric patients may have a parent stay in the room. The parent will be required to wear a lead apron to prevent radiation exposure.

After procedure:
- Drink a lot of water to flush out contrast.
- You may return to your normal activities.

Benefits:
- Other than the IV, the procedure is painless and noninvasive.
- Precise: can identify tumors, abnormal blood vessels, brain shrinkage, scar tissue, and strokes.
- Able to image bone, soft tissue, and blood vessels all at the same time.
- Takes images from sagittal (vertical) and axial (parallel) views.
- Examination is fast and simple.
- No dark tunnel.
- The machine is open.
- Donut-like opening is 27 – 30 inches.
- Can be performed if you have an implanted medical device of any kind.
- No radiation remains in your body.
- Usually no side effects.

Disadvantages:
- Delivers a relatively high dosage of radiation.
- Uncomfortable due to lying still for a long time.

Risks:
- Slight chance of cancer. The amount of radiation is variable to the scanner type (different models and manufacturers), and *repeated tests.*
- Compared to other diagnostic tests, it delivers moderate to high dose of radiation.
- Rare chance of serious allergic reactions to contrast materials that contain iodine. Radiology departments are well prepared to respond.

M.E.G. (Magnetoencephalogram)
a.k.a.
M.S.I. (Magnetic Source Imaging)

Used to identify abnormal electrical discharges that produce magnetic signals in the brain. It's a functional imaging technique that looks at brain activity, not just brain structure. In presurgical evaluation, it's used to find and map the sensory, motor, and language areas.

Preparation:
- You may be asked to stay up late the night before the test, so you're sleepy during the recording.
- If you're sedated, you'll be asked to not eat for eight hours before the test.
- Your hair should be washed and left loose.
- You can wear your own clothing during the scan considering there's no metal on them. You can wear elasticized pants or similar clothing without metal fasteners. Women are encouraged to wear sports bras.

Procedure:
- You will go into a special magnetic-free room. (The room is lined in a special metal which protects the scanner from interference that can negatively affect the scan).
- You will have three coils which are placed on a Velcro headband, attached to your head (used to determine exactly where your head is, inside the scanner).
- You will sit on a chair, which moves slowly through the scanner.
- Since you have to remain very still, a cushion might be placed around your head to help keep your head still.
- The scanner is very quiet. (You won't be able to tell when the scanner is taking pictures)!
- During the scan, you may be asked to perform a task (such as tapping your fingers or looking at pictures).
- The technologist will leave the room during the procedure but can see and talk with you through a speaker.
- *The procedure itself takes about 3 – 4 hours.*

After procedure:
- You'll leave the MEG room and will sit on a chair while the tech will use a pen to trace around your head (to make an accurate model of the shape of your head).
- There are no restrictions or special instructions.
- You're free to go home and enjoy your normal activities.

Benefits:
- Noninvasive
- Painless

Disadvantages:
- You must remain still or the test may need to be repeated.
- The procedure is considerably long.

Risks:
- The test is safe. There have been no reported complications.

P.E.T. scan
(Positron Emission Tomography)

Nuclear medicine test to *find tissue function images to see if your brain is metabolizing glucose.* The computer turns the measurements received from the scan into two or three dimensional images. The result is a colorful picture showing which parts of your brain were most active (based on the amount of glucose at use). The results are very precise breaking down the activity into a variety of colors recognizing five levels of intensity, which include low, medium high, very high, medium, low, and no activity.

Preparation:
- Fasting for a certain time prior to the procedure is required, usually for at least four hours.
- You will receive special instructions ahead of time regarding the number of hours you are to withhold food and drink.
- Your doctor will inform you regarding the use of your medications prior to the scan.
- You should not consume any caffeine or alcohol, or use tobacco for at least 24 hours prior to the procedure.

- Your doctor will give you specific instructions based on your individual situation. In addition prior to the procedure, a fasting blood sugar test may be necessary. If the level is elevated, it may be necessary to give you insulin to lower your blood sugar.

Procedure:
- You will be laid on a padded table, which slides inside the scanner.
- One or two IV lines will be started.
- The radionuclide solution will go through the IV.
- You will wait for approximately 45 – 60 minutes for the radionuclide to travel through your body until it concentrates in your brain.
- You will lie still, rest quietly, and avoid significant movement or talking.
- After the solution has been absorbed, the table will move slowly into the donut-like scanner (much like the CT scan machine).
- You must lie still during the test.
- You will be able to communicate with the technician.
- You'll hear whirring and clicking sounds. (Some machines are louder than others).
- The actual test ranges from 30 – 45 minutes (not including the radionuclide concentration time).
- *The approximate length of time for the test including the radionuclide injection and positioning is 1 ½ hours.*

After procedure:
- The technician checks the IV site for signs of redness or swelling.
- The scan itself is painless but lying still for a long time may cause some discomfort.
- You can resume your normal activities.
- If you notice any pain, redness, and/or swelling at the IV site after you return home following the procedure, you should notify your doctor.
- Although it's short-lived, the radionuclide should be flushed out of your system by drinking plenty of fluids and emptying your bladder frequently for up to 48 hours.

Benefits:
- The focus of the seizures are located for some patients

- An effective way to examine the chemical activity in your brain.
- Accurately assesses sites in the brain for delicate surgery.
- Radiation exposure is low.
- Overall test is safe.

Disadvantages:
- Radiotracer must be used.
- Invasive.
- You must wait 45 – 60 minutes for the radiotracer to concentrate in your brain before test starts.
- Lying still for a long time may cause some discomfort.

Risks:
- Allergic reactions from the radiotracer may occur. However, they are extremely rare.

S.P.E.C.T.
(single photon emission computed tomography)

Large circular device, which contains a special camera that detects the amount of radioactive tracer absorbed by your body. Images concentrate at the seizure region, which can help identify the location of the seizures and assist doctors concerning the blood flow to your brain tissue. Analyzing blood flow to your brain may help determine how specific areas are functioning. For example, blood flow increases to an area of the brain in people with epilepsy when on the other hand a person without epilepsy shows a decreased blood flow. The pictures go to a computer that uses the information to create 3-D images.

Preparation:
- You can wear your own clothing during the scan considering there's no metal on them. You can wear elasticized sweat pants or similar clothing without metal fasteners. Women are encouraged to wear sports bras.
- Plan to stay between 1 – 2 hours.
- There are no restrictions on what you can eat or drink.

Procedure:

- An IV line will be started.
- You'll receive a small amount of radioactive tracer called radiobled through an IV. (In some cases, you may inhale the substance through your nose).
- You will need to rest about 10 – 20 minutes until the tracer reaches your brain.
- Then you will lie comfortably on a table-like bed on the scanner.
- The scan will not hurt. However, you may feel uncomfortable due to lying still for an extended period.
- The machine will rotate around you. You will not be in a tube-like machine. It's comparable to a large X-ray machine over your head with just a few inches clearance. However, the sides are open so it is not as confining as many other scans.
- You will need to remain as still as possible.
- You will have a strap on your head to keep your head in the correct position.
- In some cases, you may receive a sedative before the test to help keep you more comfortable while lying still.
- *The test ranges from 30 – 90 minutes.*

After procedure:

- Once the scan is complete, you can leave.
- You should drink plenty of fluids in order to flush out any tracer left in your body.

Benefits:

- Comparable to a P.E.T. scan in providing medical information but less expensive.
- High sensitivity (picks up images clearly).
- Most of the tracer leaves your body through your urine within a few hours.
- Your body will break down the remaining radioactive tracer over the next day or two.

Disadvantages:

- You need to rest about 10 – 20 minutes before the test starts until the tracer reaches your brain.

- You may experience discomfort from lying still for a long time.
- Invasive.

Risks:
- In general, the radiation levels are similar to those you might encounter naturally in the environment over the course of a year.
- Possibility of allergic reaction to radioactive tracer.
- You may experience bleeding, pain or swelling in the particular area where the IV was inserted.
- For most people, S.P.E.C.T. scans are safe. Threats are minimal.

External E.E.G.
(*electroencephalography*)

Digital monitoring apparatus that records electrical activity in the brain through electrodes. E.e.g.s have been proven to be the most useful test in detecting seizure activity, types of seizures, amount of seizures, and localizing the area in the brain from which the seizures are originating. Approximately 10 – 15 minutes of recording results in 20 – 30 pages of paper can be bound and read like a book!

All external e.e.g.'s are prepared for, applied, and removed the same way.

Preparation:
- Eat as usual excluding tea, coffee, cola, etc. starting the night before the test.
- Take regularly scheduled medication as prescribed unless instructed by your doctor otherwise.
- Wear comfortable clothing with a loose fitting button front shirt.
- Wash hair (Do not use styling products such as conditioner, gel, and hairspray).
- Remove braids and hair extensions.

Applying e.e.g. electrodes:
- The technician will measure your head.
- A soft wax crayon is used to mark specific points on your scalp and forehead (for accurate electrode placement).

- Scalp points are rubbed with a mild abrasive cream (improves signals for quality of recording).
- Conductive gel is used on up to 25 electrodes.
- Electrodes are secured to your scalp and forehead with water-soluble glue.
- Your head will be wrapped with gauze.
- The electrodes are connected to a computer or a microcomputer in a "fanny pack", depending on the test.

Removal of electrodes:
- The technician will remove electrodes from your scalp with acetone or a similar product.
- Your skin and hair will remain intact.
- You'll need to wash any remaining glue out of your hair. (You may need more acetone to remove any remaining glue).
- There may be mild irritation where electrodes were placed.
- If medication was reduced for the test, your doctor may have further instructions.

Standard E.E.G.

Procedure:
- You will be positioned on a padded bed, table or comfortable chair.
- You will lie or sit still and can not talk unless absolutely necessary.
- You may be asked to have your eyes open. Then, later asked to keep them closed.
- You may be asked to breathe deeply and rapidly.
- If you're prone to photogenic seizures, a flashing light may be used in front of you.
- *Test takes approximately one hour.*

After procedure:
- Typically, you can return to your regular activities unless otherwise instructed by your doctor.

Benefits:
- The procedure is painless and noninvasive.
- No medication reduction or withdrawal is necessary.

- Records subtle seizures unrecognized by you.
- Does not require hospitalization.

Disadvantages:
- Captures limited amount of information.

Risks:
- The procedure is safe. There have been no negative reports.

Sleep Deprived

This procedure is similar to a standard e.e.g. but is more appropriate for children and patients with relatively frequent seizure activity, (at least three seizures per week). Sleep often brings out abnormalities that may not be seen in the awake, state. Only 50% of abnormalities may be seen in the awake, state and may increase to 85% in the asleep, state. To increase the chance of recording seizures, sleep deprivation is required for this test. Sleep deprivation may be defined as a few hours less than the usual amount of sleep. It's also often used to *activate seizures or abnormal activity* otherwise not seen.

Procedure:
- It's important to relax.
- You may *be asked to look at light that flashes at different rates.*
- *You may be asked to breath deeply and rapidly (*hyperventilate*).*
- *You may be asked to sleep.*
- *The test will take about 1 ½ – 2 hours.*

After procedure:
- You should have someone drive you home.
- You can return to your regular activities unless otherwise instructed by your doctor.

Benefits:
- More convenient than inpatient e.e.g.
- Stressing the brain may give additional diagnostic information.
- The procedure is painless and noninvasive.
- Helps determine if sleep deprivation is the cause of seizures.
- Nurses and doctors are available.

Disadvantages:
- Captures limited amount of information.
- You must be kept awake prior to test.
- The test is considerably long.

Risks:
- The procedure is safe. No reports have proven otherwise.

Ambulatory E.E.G. *a.k.a.* A.E.E.G.

If you are unable to have a v.e.e.g., the ambulatory e.e.g. enables your doctor to observe your brain's activity over a prolonged period of time. Electrode wires are connected to a box which carries a micro-computer that is stored in a "fanny pack" on a shoulder strap.

Procedure:
- After the electrodes are attached to your scalp they'll be plugged into a microcomputer and put in a "fanny pack."
- You may go home or wherever else you wish to be.
- You'll keep the "fanny pack" on at all times which will have an "event" button attached to it.
- You'll take your medications as prescribed unless otherwise instructed by your doctor.
- You'll sleep with the fanny pack which will remain attached to the microcomputer.
- You'll push the "event" button every time you:
  - ► Feel a sensation which did not progress into a seizure.
  - ► Experience an aura.
  - ► Have a seizure if you're conscious, and after the seizure.
- You'll keep a log to record specific details.

After procedure:
- You can enjoy your regular activities unless otherwise instructed by your doctor.

Benefits:
- Procedure is painless and noninvasive.
- Records continuously for up to 72 hours.

- No medication reduction or withdrawal.
- Less expensive than inpatient e.e.g.
- Provides more information than a standard e.e.g.
- Recognizes all seizure types.
- Records subtle seizures unrecognized by you.
- Seizure activity will show during sleep.
- Does not require hospitalization.

Disadvantages:
- No video monitoring.
- No nurse to assist you during or after a seizure.
- No technician to fix loose wires.
- Less opportunity to catch seizure activity.

Risks:
- The procedure is safe. There have been no claims to suggest otherwise.

V.E.E.G.
(Video E.E.G. Monitoring)

Prolonged inpatient recordings provide more data than the outpatient e.e.g. Video monitoring is essential along with an e.e.g. because together they provide visualization of the actual events. The signals from both the video and e.e.g. are transmitted to a control room where the e.e.g. is reformatted and conducted to a video monitor. They are displayed together for online observation. Both are recorded on videotape. The e.e.g. may be recorded on paper and/or on a compact disc.

As a general rule this test should be performed on any patient who continues to have frequent seizures despite therapeutic treatment. The inpatient video e.e.g. is the most valuable test in the beginning of your search for the treatment specifically designed for you.

Procedure:
- After electrodes have been attached you'll go to your room in the E.C.U.

- The transmitter in the "fanny pack" will be connected to the wall outlet through the coaxial cable.
- You'll wear the "fanny pack" with the e.e.g. transmitter connected to a wall outlet at all times.
- A wall mount video camera provides continuous observation.
- For monitoring purposes only, your medication might be reduced to allow a seizure to occur.
- You will have two alarm buttons. One for the nurse and the other for the seizure "event" button.
- You can carry out normal activities such as watch television, talk, and nap.
- You can move around your room freely but will be encouraged to stay in video range.
- You will be viewed by a monitor at the nurses' station at all times.
- Showers are allowed. A nurse or assistant will remove the fanny pack, and wrap your head with a water proof cover.
- Some facilities allow access to a recreation room. If so, the coaxial cable will be unplugged from your room and plugged into a wall outlet specifically labeled for you to continue recording in the recreation room.
- *The hospital stay is typically 3 – 4 days.*

For the hospital stay:
- Take a loose fitting *head wrap, such as a bandanna* (for appearance purpose only)!
- Take your own pillow (if you desire, and if facility allows).
- Children can take a stuffed animal, blanket, or any other item(s) that comforts them.
- Take items to help pass the time. (Check with facility regarding electronic devices).

After procedure:
- You may return to your daily activities unless otherwise instructed by your doctor.

Benefits:
- Less chance of injury during seizure.
- Allows for sleep-invoked seizures.
- The procedure is noninvasive and painless.

- Nurses available for immediate care.
- Neurologist/epileptologist is available.
- Finds amount of seizure activity.
- Finds subtle unnoticed seizures.
- Recognizes all seizure types.
- Reasonable amount of time to record seizures.
- Video monitoring is available for additional information.
- Communication with medical staff.
- Diagnosis can be made definitely in nearly all cases.
- Determines seizures focal areas (in most cases).
- Seizures can be recorded during sleep (increases possibility of recording nocturnal seizures).

Disadvantages:
- Requires hospitalization.
- May not offer precise information. (if necessary for surgical candidates).

Risks:
- Skin irritation or redness may be present at the locations where the electrodes were placed.
- The test is safe. There have been no reported complaints.

Intracranial E.E.G.

Intracranial e.e.g. monitoring (subdural and depth) provides additional information *necessary* for the neurologist and neurosurgeon when surgery is considered. They are used to record electrical activity directly from the brain without interference from the scalp and skull. Intracranial e.e.g.'s are sometimes needed to map the specific areas from which the seizures begin. Whether subdural or depth electrodes are used depends on findings of the noninvasive studies (standard e.e.g., v.e.e.g., etc.). Subdural and depth electrodes are *very* similar. Depth electrodes are inserted in your brain where subdural electrodes are laid on your brain.

Expect the following tests prior to implantation surgery for both depth and subdural electrodes:
- Blood work
- CT/CAT scan

- E.E.G.
- M.R.I.
- P.E.T. scan
- S.P.E.C.T.
- Wada

Preparation prior to surgery for both depth and subdural electrodes:
- You'll refrain from eating and drinking according to your doctor's instructions.
- The night before surgery, you'll wash your entire body with Hibiclens (presurgical antiseptic antimicrobial skin cleanser).
- Blood work will be taken.
- You'll have a brief physical to check your pulse, blood pressure, and temperature.
- The nurse will review your paperwork to confirm information.
- An IV line will be started.
- You'll be taken to the operating room.
- You'll be placed asleep under general anesthesia.

Intracranial e.e.g. surgeries are extremely complex, and very similar. The steps described below are very simplistic. The intention is to give you a basic idea of what happens during the surgeries. Keep in mind, the technique for each may be different from one facility to another due to neurosurgeon and/or facility preference.

Surgery to implant electrodes:
- Your head will be shaved.
- Electrode placement is performed with either a frameless system or a stereotactic head frame.
- An MRI may be taken.
- The neurosurgeon will make several burr holes in your skull.
- The electrodes will be strategically implanted *in* (depth) or placed *on* (subdural) your brain.
- The electrodes will be inserted through the burr holes.
- They'll be connected to a transmitter in a "fanny pack."
- Your head will be wrapped in a bandage for protection and padding.
- You'll be moved to the recovery room.
- *The surgery may take up to six hours.*

Procedure:

- You will be taken to your E.C.U. room.
- The transmitter in the "fanny pack" will be connected to the wall outlet through the coaxial cable.
- You'll wear a "fanny pack" with the e.e.g. transmitter connected to a wall outlet at all times.
- A wall mount video camera provides continuous observation.
- You will have two alarm buttons. One for the nurse and the other for the seizure "event" button.
- You can carry out normal activities such as watch television, talk, and nap.
- You will be viewed by a monitor at the nurses' station at all times.
- Continuous v.e.e.g. testing is performed.
- Antiepileptic medications might be tapered.
- *The electrodes may be left in for 1 – 2 weeks depending on the number or seizures you have.*

Depth Electrodes

After electrode procedure:

- You will return to surgery.
- The electrodes will be removed.
- If a focal area or areas of seizure activity is found, and will not affect important areas of your brain (such as speech and motor functions), you will have a resection.
- *You may be hospitalized up to ten days, depending on the number of seizures you have.*

Benefits:

- Decreases operative time and potential risks of brain surgery.
- Useful for precisely mapping the origin of the seizures.
- Determines if there is more than one focal point for seizure onset.
- Allows for mapping of critical brain areas.
- Determines if the speech center is near the seizure focus.
- Electrodes are removed during the same operation as the lobectomy.
- Does not require a large opening in your skull.

- Less likely than subdural electrodes to cause infection or brain swelling.
- Correctly identifies temporal lobe seizures more often than subdural electrodes.

Disadvantages:
- Identifies temporal lobe seizures less often than depth electrodes.
- The procedure is invasive and painful.
- Requires hospitalization.

Risks:
- Infection
- Stroke
- Brain bleeding
- Brain swelling

Subdural Electrodes

There are two types of subdural electrodes, strip and grid. Many centers use grid in combination with strip electrodes.

Subdural strip Six to eight contact points are used to record electrical activity from your brain. They lay on the *surface* of the brain rather than in the brain tissue. Burr holes may be drilled in the skull in order to place them.

Subdural grid Up to 64 contact points are used to record the brain's electrical activity. A portion of the skull is temporarily removed (craniotomy) in order to place the grid. It's placed on the surface of the brain.

After procedure:
- If a focal area or areas of seizure activity is found, and will not affect essential areas of your brain, (such as speech and motor functions), you will return to surgery for a lobectomy.
- The electrodes will be removed first.
- The resection will be performed.

- *You may be hospitalized up to ten days, depending on the number of seizures you have.*

Benefits:
- Decreases operative time.
- Wires do not penetrate the brain.
- Decreases potential risks of brain surgery.
- Useful for precisely mapping the origin of the seizure.
- Allows for brain mapping of critical brain areas.
- Determines if speech center is near the seizure focus.
- Wires are removed during same operation as resection.
- Less likely than subdural electrodes to cause infection or brain swelling.

Disadvantages:
- Identifies and lateralizes temporal lobe seizures less   often than depth electrodes.
- Considerable disadvantages depend on technique used.
- Painful and invasive.
- Requires hospitalization.

Risks:
- Infection
- Stroke
- Brain bleeding
- Brain swelling

M. R. I.

MRI (Magnetic Resonance Imaging) Procedure using powerful magnets and radio waves to construct clear, detailed pictures of brain tissue. People with cardiac pacemakers will not be scanned and should never enter the MRI area. People with metallic objects in their bodies such as inner ear (cochlear) implants, brain aneurysm clips, some artificial heart valves, older vascular stents, and recently placed artificial joints should also not enter the MRI area, because the strong magnetic fields can displace or disrupt their action. The technologist will provide you with a questionnaire, which lists the potentially dangerous items.

Traditional Closed
(whole body)

Narrow tube-like machine about two feet in diameter and six to eight feet long. The moveable bed goes into, the cylinder-shaped machine which is surrounded by a circular magnet. During a closed M.R.I., you are fully surrounded by the tunnel.

Preparation:
- Unless otherwise instructed, you may follow your regular daily routine and take your medications as usual.
- Avoid caffeinated beverages.
- Keep jewelry at home.
- If you suffer from claustrophobia, you may request a mild sedative to take in advance.
- You can wear your own clothing during the scan considering there's no metal on them. You can wear elasticized sweat pants. Women are encouraged to wear sports bras. Otherwise a hospital gown may be recommended.

Procedure:
- You will be positioned on a movable bed-like table.
- An IV line will be started.
- Straps will be used to help you remain still and maintain the correct position during imaging.
- Small devices that contain coils for sending and receiving radio waves may be placed around your head.
- Contrast material will be administered through the IV.
- It's normal to feel a warm and flushing sensation for a minute or two from the contrast material.
- Once you have received all the contrast, you will be moved into the tunnel.
- You will not feel the radio waves or the magnetic field.
- The table may be cold but you can request a blanket.

- During the test, the machine produces a loud thumping noise, mimicking a jackhammer. You will be given earplugs to mask the noise of the machine.
- Straps may be placed across your head to prevent movement and remain in the correct position.
- The technologist will be able to see you during the scan. You will be able to communicate with them through an intercom system inside the scanner. Some MRI scanners are equipped with televisions and special headphones to help pass the examination time.
- *The test ranges from 30 – 45 minutes.*

After the Procedure:
- If you have not been sedated, no recovery period is necessary.
- If you have been sedated, you will need someone to drive you home.
- You can resume your normal diet, activity, and medications immediately after the test.
- Drink a lot of water to flush the contrast out of your system.

Benefits:
- No ionizing radiation.
- Contrast materials have a very low incidence of side effects.
- Rare documented allergic reactions.
- No potential for medical related complications.
- Helps doctor evaluate the structures of your brain.
- Provides functional information.
- Detects abnormalities hidden by bone structures obscured by other imaging methods.
- Provides best imaging of all MRI machines.
- Performed on an outpatient basis.

Disadvantages:
- May experience claustrophobia.
- Must remain extremely still for extended period of time.

Risks:
- Rare possibility of allergic side effects from contrast which includes itchy watery eyes.
- Test is very safe.

Short-bore
(open)

Designed so the magnet will not surround you. These units are especially helpful for examining patients who are claustrophobic and those who are obese. However, they may not provide the same image quality as traditional systems. They cannot be used for certain types of scans.

Preparation:
- Unless you are otherwise instructed, you may follow your regular daily routine and take your medications as usual.
- Avoid caffeinated beverages.
- You can wear your own clothing during the scan considering there's no metal on them. You can wear elasticized sweat pants or similar clothing without metal fasteners. Women are encouraged to wear sports bras.
- Keep all jewelry at home.
- If you have difficulty lying still, and/or are very anxious, you may be given a sedative.

Procedure:
- You'll lie on a flat moveable table.
- An IV line will be started.
- A contrast dye will be administered through the IV.
- When the contrast material is injected, it is normal to feel a cool and flushing sensation for a minute or two.
- You'll be positioned on a moveable bed-like table with your head cradled on a headrest and your arms at your sides.
- Straps will be used to help you maintain the correct position during imaging.
- The technologist may place small lifesaver-looking markers on your forehead, face or behind your ear (if test is for surgery).
- Once positioned, you must remain still.
- The table will slowly move into the "donut hole" machine.
- The technologist will stay in constant contact with you, and you may also stay in contact with the technologist.
- When the test starts, you will hear clicking then thumping sounds.
- *The test ranges from 20 –35 minutes.*

After procedure:
- No recovery period is necessary.
- You can go home after the test is completed.
- If you have been sedated, you will need someone to drive you home.
- You can resume your normal diet, activity, and medications immediately after the test.
- Drink a lot of water to flush the contrast out of your system.

Benefits:
- Wide open design.
- No dark tunnel.
- Accommodates obese and claustrophobic patients.
- Reduced noise compared to a closed MRI.
- Quality images.
- More face space and elbow room compared to closed MRI.
- Shorter exams than closed MRI.
- No ionizing radiation.
- Results more reliable than Wada.
- Contrast materials have a very low incidence of side effects.
- No potential for medical related complications.
- Has ability to image in any direction.
- Provides much more specificity.
- Defines tissue characteristics which provide detailed information.
- Performed on an outpatient basis.
- Possesses superior soft tissue imaging.
- Great substitute for Wada study due to its ability to see real time activity in the brain.
- Test is very safe.

Disadvantages:
- Contrast must be used.

Risks:
- No health risks associated with the magnetic field or the radio waves.
- Rare possibility of allergic side effects from contrast which includes itchy watery eyes.

F.M.R.I.
(Functional)

Measures your brain's activity. It detects changes in blood flow rather than the quantity of a radioactive tracer which in turn detects abnormalities. When a particular part in your brain experiences increased activity, there is a sudden rush of blood flow. Therefore, the scan can detect active sites in the brain in real time.

Preparation:
- Unless you are otherwise instructed, you may follow your regular daily routine and take your medications as usual.
- If you have difficulty lying still, and/or are very anxious you may be given a sedative.
- Avoid caffeinated beverages.
- You can wear your own clothing during the scan considering there's no metal on them. You can wear elasticized sweat pants or similar clothing without metal fasteners. Women are encouraged to wear sports bras.

Procedure:
- You'll be given earplugs to mask the noise of the machine.
- You'll be laid on a flat moveable table.
- An IV line will be started and the contrast will be administered.
- Your head will be placed in a brace which may include a mask.
- You may be given special goggles and/or earphones to wear.
- Straps may be used to help you remain still and in the correct position.
- You'll be moved headfirst into the machine.
- During scanning, you'll be asked to perform tasks (such as touch your thumb to your fingers, and answer simple questions).
- *The test is typically completed in 45 minutes.*

After procedure:
- No recovery period is necessary.
- You can go home after the test is completed.
- If you have been sedated, you will need someone to drive you home.

- You should drink a lot of water to flush the contrast out of your system.
- You can resume your normal diet, activity, and medications immediately after the test.

Benefits:
- Ionizing radiation is not used.
- Contrast materials have a very low incidence of side effects.
- Results more reliable than Wada.
- No potential for medical related complications.
- Has ability to image in any direction.
- Provides much more specificity.
- Defines tissue characteristics which provide useful information.
- Performed on an outpatient basis.
- Possesses superior soft tissue imaging.
- Generates a series of images shown in thin "slices."
- Due to its ability to see real time activity in the brain it's a great substitute for the Wada study.

Disadvantages:
- A contrast must be used.

Risks:
- MRI is very safe.
- Rare possibility of allergic side effects from contrast.

Stand-up

Although the stand-up MRI exists, it's not practical for brain images. The major purpose is to allow the patient to bear weight on the body's pathology by simply standing up. This feature is important in obtaining images of the spine and joints in positions of normal stress. It's especially useful in determining the underlying cause of pain.

Other Tests

Medical History Reviewing your detailed medical history including symptoms and duration of the seizures is an important issue in the process to determine if you have epilepsy. The doctor will ask you questions about the seizures and any past illnesses or other symptoms you had. Since people who suffer from seizures do not often remember what happened, caregivers, family, and friends accounts of the seizures are vital for this evaluation may be requested for this particular test.

Developmental, Neurological, and Behavioral Tests Measures motor abilities, behavior, and intellectual capacity to determine how the epilepsy is affecting you. These tests can also provide clues about what kind of epilepsy you have.

Neuropsychological Testing Evaluates your current level of brain functioning, including memory, visual, verbal, attention, mood, language, personality, and thought process that might correlate with diagnostic imaging and e.e.g.

Psychiatric evaluation Undergoing surgery for epilepsy is a long and difficult process. A psychiatric evaluation helps you develop reasonable goals and expectations, as well as prepare you for surgery and recovery aspects.

Visual field evaluation Measures your peripheral side view field of vision. You will hold your head still while looking at an object in front or beside you.

WADA
(intracarotid amytal test)

A two part test named after Japanese doctor, *Juhn Wada*. The Wada is only used for surgical purposes, as far as epilepsy is concerned. The purpose of the test is to mimic the effects of surgery. Both sides of your brain are connected and always working together. During the Wada test however, one side of your brain is "put to sleep" in order to see if the other can talk and remember! That is the whole basis of the test. The origin of the test was to determine the language dominant side of the brain. Then a modification was to detect which side of the brain has better memory.

It requires participation of a large medical team including a radiologist, radiologic technologists, nurses, neuropsychologists, and e.e.g. technologist. It works hand in hand with an angiogram, which is directly prior to the Wada. It looks at the blood flow within your brain to make sure there are no obstacles to keep from performing the Wada safely.

Your doctor may request a blood test prior to the procedure to determine how long it takes your blood to clot. Since the Wada is back to back with the angiogram, you need to schedule a physical exam within 30 days of the scheduled Wada.

Before scheduling the angiogram, notify your doctor if you:
- Had an adverse reaction to any contrast dye.
- Are allergic to anesthetics, iodine, latex, medications, seafood, tape.
- Take herbal supplements, over the counter and/or prescription medications.
- Have a history of bleeding disorders.
- Are taking an anticoagulant (blood-thinning) medication.
- Are taking aspirin and/or ibuprofen.
- Are taking medications that affect blood clotting.

It may be necessary to stop some medications prior to the procedure. After you schedule the procedure, make plans to have someone drive you home.

Preparation:
- Do not eat or drink anything after midnight the night before the test.
- Continue taking presently scheduled prescriptions, unless otherwise instructed by your doctor.
- Take a sedative provided by the facility, if you feel it's necessary.
- Make arrangements to get a ride home.
- Make a preparation to stay over night (unlikely).

Part One:
- Remove all clothing and jewelry. *You'll be provided with a patient gown.*
- Both the technologist and radiologist will stay by your side.

- You'll be positioned on an X-ray table.
- An EKG (disc–like stickers with wires, no needles) will be attached to your chest strictly for monitoring.
- The radiologist will check your pulse around the catheter site, usually in the groin, and will mark it with a pen or marker.
- A local anesthetic (numbing solution) will be used, where the incision will be made.
- The catheter will be inserted through the incision and placed in the carotid artery.
- The catheter will be directed to the right or left carotid artery in your neck.
- Once the catheter is inserted, an X-ray is taken to verify the location.
- After you are properly placed on the exam table, your head will be positioned in the desired position.
- You will be immobilized with straps across your forehead.
- The contrast dye will be administered through the catheter.
- Your mouth may get dry.
- You may feel a flushing sensation a salty or metallic taste, a brief headache, and nausea (usually last only a few moments).
- After the contrast dye is administered, a series of X-rays are taken.
- There may be one or more injections of contrast dye through the catheter.
- The catheter stays in place for the Wada test.
- After minimal bleeding stops at the site, a dressing is applied.
- Pressure is placed over the site for a period of time (to avoid bleeding and clotting).

Part Two:
- Your head will be placed in a plastic "ring" and held into place with straps in order to keep it in the position and hold it still.
- Heart monitor patches will stay on your chest from the angiogram.
- The catheter will remain in place from the angiogram and directed towards the carotid arteries. (Most patients do not feel the movement of the catheter).
- The catheter is gently guided to its destination.
- Sodium amobarbital is injected through the catheter.
- The injection will cause one side of your brain (the side of the injection) to "go to sleep" for a few minutes.

- Once the doctors are sure it's asleep, a neuropsychologist shows you objects and pictures.
- The alert side of the brain tries to recognize and remember what it sees.
- After just a few minutes, the sodium amobarbital wears off.
- The side that was asleep starts to wake up.
- Once both sides of your brain are fully awake, the neuropsychologist will ask for details to what you saw.
- If you do not remember what you saw, items are shown again one at a time.
- You are asked if you saw each one.
- Your responses will be recorded word-for-word.
- The catheter is then removed.
- A new angiogram is done on the other side of your brain.
- After a delay, the other side of your brain is "put to sleep."
- The "awake," side (which was "asleep" before) tries to recognize and remember what it sees.
- Then the "asleep," side goes through the same visual test.
- Once both sides are awake, you will be asked what was shown the second time.
- The duration of the Wada study can vary between medical facilities. Some have a 30–60 minute delay *between injections*.
- The catheter will be removed immediately after the last memory test. No stitches will be necessary.
- The Wada is minimally uncomfortable. There is no significant pain to fear. Actually, you will probably find this particular test amusing during the memory part!
- *The test in its entirety varies between facilities, and ranges from 30 – 60 minutes.*

After procedure:
- You will be on bed rest with bathroom privileges for the remainder of the day.
- The nurses and doctors will be checking the pulse in your legs where the catheters were inserted and check under the dressings.
- Sensory checks will also be done throughout the day.
- If the puncture is checked and stable and no complications arise, you will be discharged the same day.

- You are to avoid strenuous activity for at least 24 – 48 hours after the procedure.

Benefits:
- Confirms which side of the brain stores memory.
- Replaces the option of memory testing while awake during brain surgeries.

Disadvantage:
- The procedure is invasive and minimally painful.
- You have restrictions for 2 – 3 days after the procedure.

Risks:
- Stroke (1% chance) and greater chance if you are older or have atherosclerosis or a history of high cholesterol. Neither poses an extreme threat.
- Bleeding
- Infection

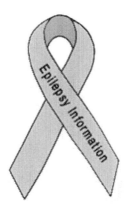

Seizure Types and Triggers

The brain runs on chemical and electrical signals. A seizure is an electrical storm in the brain. Seizures can cause involuntary changes in body movement, function, sensation, awareness, and behavior. Symptoms experienced during a seizure depend on where the disturbance in electrical activity occurs.

There are many variables for seizure activity. The numerous epileptic seizure types are most commonly defined and grouped according to a scheme proposed by the International League against Epilepsy (ILAE). Distinguishing between seizure types is important since different types of seizures may have different causes, prognosis, and treatments.

Aura is a type of simple partial seizure, which sometimes signals the onset of a generalized or complex partial seizure.

Possible Characteristics:
- Déjà vu
- Dizziness
- Odors
- Sounds
- Stomach discomfort

- Uneasiness/fear
- Visual illusions or misconceptions
- Warm fuzzy feeling
- Feeling of slow motion

Febrile Seizures are related to high fevers in babies and children, usually under age five. Most children who have a febrile seizure do not develop epilepsy.

Characteristics:
- Body, arms, and legs are stiff; and slowly jerking violently
- Eyes roll up
- Not breathing well (may turn blue)
- Not responding
- Not crying

Pseudo/Non-epileptic Psychological, non-epileptic seizure (NES) may be related to physical illness, psychiatric disorder or emotional attacks.

Characteristics:
- There is a sudden disruptive change in behavior.
- Resembles epileptic seizures but has no physiological change in the brain.
- The brain activity is normal.

Primary Generalized Epilepsy

Primary generalized epilepsy is a type of epilepsy, which occurs when electrical discharges begin in both sides of the brain at the same time.

Absence Formerly known as petit mal. This seizure speaks for itself!

Characteristics:
- Abrupt onset
- Brief duration
- Vacant staring (much like daydreaming)

- Begins and ends abruptly
- Impairment lifts
- Person returns to previous activity
- No after effect

Atonic Also known as, "drop attacks" or "drop seizures." Atonic means "without tone." Another name is *"akinetic"* which means "without movement." Atonic seizures typically begin in childhood.

Characteristics:
- Eyelids may droop
- Fall suddenly
- Head drops suddenly
- No change in awareness
- Lose strength in legs
- Objects fall from hands
- Sudden loss of muscle tone

Atypical absence means unusual or not typical. They usually begin in childhood. They are easily controlled with medication. Approximately 75 percent of children outgrow them. The behavior can be hard to distinguish from the person's usual behavior like daydreaming, especially in those with cognitive mental processes of perceiving, thinking, and remembering. Unlike other absence seizures, these seizures usually cannot be produced by rapid breathing.

Characteristics:
- Brief automatic movements of the mouth or hands (sometimes).
- Eye blinking (sometimes).
- Slight jerking movements of the lips may occur.
- Brief myoclonic jerking of the eyelids.
- Brief myoclonic jerking of the facial muscles.
- Somewhat responsive.
- Staring (as in absence seizures).
- Usually lasts less than 30 seconds.

Clonic "Clonus" means rapidly alternating contraction and relaxation of a muscle. The movements cannot be stopped by restraining or repositioning the arms or legs. Clonic seizures are rare. They can occur at various ages requiring prolonged treatment. They also occur in newborns but disappear on their own within a brief time.

Characteristics:
- Jerking movements (of the arms and legs involving muscles on both sides of the body).
- Repeated jerking.
- Length varies.

Myoclonic "Myo" means muscle. "Clonus" means rapidly alternating contraction and relaxation of a muscle.

Characteristics:
- Brief jerks of muscle group, usually no longer than a second or two, could be just one. (Sometimes many will occur within a short time).
- Hiccups or sudden jerk that may awaken the person presently while fall asleep (normal).
- May or may not be associated with loss of consciousness, abnormal movements or behavior.

Status epilepticus is a prolonged seizure or more than one seizure, without a normal break in between. It's a medical emergency and requires emergency treatment immediately.

Characteristics:
- Prolonged seizure lasts longer than 30 minutes.
- Series of repeated seizures.
- Continuous state of seizure activity.
- May occur in almost any seizure type.

Tonic Usually involves all or most of the brain, affecting both sides of the body. They can occur in anyone and affects both children and adults.

Characteristics:
- Change in behavior.
- Falls if standing when the seizure starts.

- Occurs while awake.
- Sudden whole body stiffening.
- Usually lasts less than 20 seconds.

Tonic-clonic Formerly known as "grand mal" or convulsion is an electrical discharge, which involves all or most of the brain. They can usually be controlled by (AED) antiepileptic drugs.

Characteristics:
- Falling
- Loss of consciousness
- Jerking
- Stiffening
- Air is forced past the vocal cords causing a cry or groan.
- All the muscles stiffen (tonic).
- Arms and legs jerk rapidly and rhythmically (clonic).
- Bending and relaxing at the elbows, hips, and knees.
- Bladder or bowel control sometimes lost.
- May turn blue in the face.
- Cheek or tongue may be bitten.
- Consciousness returns slowly (may be drowsy, confused, agitated, depressed).
- Generally lasts one to three minutes.

Partial

Partial seizures begin with an electrical discharge in one limited area of the brain (focal onset). Depending on where they start and which parts of the brain they involve, they may alter consciousness or awareness. They are the most common type of seizures experienced by people with epilepsy.

Characteristics:
- Remain alert.
- Remember what happened.
- May be tired and confused.
- May not return to "normal" for up to 15 minutes.

Complex partial means awareness is altered. They were once known as psychomotor seizures.

Characteristics:
- Begin with "funny" feeling or emotion (sometimes without warning).
- Blank stares.
- Performs automatic unconscious repeated movements such as lip smacking, pulling on clothes, wandering around aimlessly.
- Usually lasts between 30 seconds to two minutes.
- Awareness is altered or lost.
- May be confused and tired for 15 minutes after the seizure.
- May not feel fully "normal" for hours after the seizure.
- Inability to speak, understand and respond.

Simple Partial

Simple partial seizures affect a small area of the brain. A person suffering from simple partial seizures remain aware. Each seizure can be exceptionally different from one person to another as well as one seizure to another. They are separated by three different classifications, which include motor, sensory, and psychic.

Motor: The following characteristics are not all inclusive. Each individual experiences different sensations.

Characteristics:
- Abnormal movements such as jerking of a finger or stiffening of part of the body.
- Movements may spread, either staying on one side of the body or extending to both sides.
- Weakness.
- Speech is affected.
- Outbursts of laughter.
- Automatic hand movements.
- May not be aware of movements.

Sensory: Smell, see or taste things that are not there.

Characteristics:

- Changes in heart rate, breathing or goose bumps.
- Changes in any one of the senses.
- Experience illusions.
- Distortions of true sensations.
- Feel sensation of numbness.
- Feel sensation of pins and needles.
- Hallucinations (see things that do not exist).
- Hear clicking, ringing, person's voice (all nonexistent).
- Painful.
- Sensation of floating or spinning in space.
- Smell nonexistent things.
- Strange unpleasant feeling in stomach, chest, head.
- Taste nonexistent things.

Psychic: Change how the person thinks, feels or experiences things.

Characteristics:

- Déjà vu (things feel familiar but are new).
- Feeling as though they're outside of their body.
- Trouble with memory.
- Garbled speech.
- Inability to find the right word.
- Trouble understanding spoken and/or written language.
- Sudden fear, (often misdiagnosed for panic attacks) depression, and happiness with no outside reason.

Common Seizure Triggers

- Alcohol consumption
- Anxiety
- Non compliance with medications
- Caffeine
- Emotional stress
- Exhaustion
- Flashing or bright lights (photosensitive seizures)
- Hormonal fluctuation
- Illegal drugs

- Medical illness
- Menstruation
- Missed medication doses
- Environment/overheated (dress in layers so you can always remove a layer. Keep cold liquids available, (preferably water)
- Over the counter medications (Always check with your epileptologist before taking over the counter medications)
- Physical stress
- Poor eating habits (such as missing meals)
- Prescription medications (particularly those written by a doctor other than your epileptologist)
- Sleep deprivation (Adequate sleep is at least eight hours a night)
- Smoking
- Stress
- Artificial sweeteners
- Transition between sleep and awakening
- Head trauma
- Central nervous system infections
- Fever
- Changes in blood sugar
- Food additive, MSG

Seizure First Aid

Seizure first aid is necessary to learn, and is very simple! If your family and friends do not already know it, you need to stress how important it is, and encourage them to learn it now! It can keep you safe until the seizure stops naturally, which in turn reduces fear and stress. As silly as it may seem, it is just as important for you to know how to respond to a seizure. After all, you may meet other people with epilepsy at a local epilepsy event. You could be put on the spot, and may need to know what to do and react fast. It's equally as important for the public to know how to respond to seizures. If you know what to do, you can teach others.

- Stay calm.
- Reassure other people who may be nearby.

- Help but do not force the person to lie down.
- Don't hold them down or try to stop their movements. (You could seriously injure the person you're trying to help).
- Don't place any object into their mouth or try to force it open. (Efforts to hold their tongue down can injure their gums, teeth, and jaw).
- Protect their head. (This includes removing their glasses; and may mean going to the extreme of removing an article of your clothing or shoes to place under their head).
- Look for hazardous items and clear the area. If necessary, move the person, (if not possible to clear the area or move the person, put something in the way of the hazard which may even include putting yourself between the person and the hazard).
- Loosen anything around their neck that may restrict their breathing, such as a tie, buttoned or zipped up clothing.
- Assist them gently onto their side.
- Don't attempt CPR, unless they do not start breathing again *after* the seizure has stopped.
- Observe the event carefully so you'll be able to describe the details.
- Note the time the seizure started and duration.
- Stay with the person until the seizure ends naturally.
- Be friendly and reassuring as they become conscious. Explain to them that they just had a seizure.
- Don't give them anything to put in their mouth or let them go anywhere, until they can prove they are fully coherent by answering simple questions such as "Where are you?" What year is it? What color is my shirt? (Ask easy questions in which everyone would be capable of answering).

Seek medical help if:
- Seizure lasts longer than five minutes.
- Seizure repeats without full recovery.
- They are injured.
- It is their first seizure.
- If they do not have possession of medical alert identification such as bracelet, key chain, wallet card, etc.
- She is pregnant.

Keep in mind:

- Seizures *usually* last only a few minutes.
- They *usually* do not require medical attention.
- The person may not be aware of their actions during and after the seizure.
- They may or may not be able to hear you.
- Agitation or violent behavior during or after a seizure is common.
- Trying to restrain or grabbing a hold of them is likely to make them agitated and may trigger an instinctive aggressive response.
- Rolling them onto their side enables saliva to flow from their mouth, helping to ensure an open-air passage.
- Comfort and reassure them during and after the seizure.
- Assist them in reorienting themselves.
- They may need to rest or sleep.
- Stay with them so they will not wander.
- Talk to them with a calm voice.
- You cannot stop someone from having a seizure.

Seizure First Aid Made Easy

Seizure first aid may seem overwhelming to some people. But once they learn the steps in detail, they can be easier to remember by using acronyms. Since acronyms are brief, their intent is to help remember the details not replace them:

If you have a **plan** you will be able **to help**.

During the Seizure:
Protect their head.
Look/loosen: Look around for hazardous items. Loosen anything around their neck.
Assist them onto their side.
Nothing/never/nowhere: Nothing in their mouth. Never hold them down. Nowhere until they're alert. _Use the proof of coherence questions, "Where are you?" "What year is it?" What color is my shirt?_

Time, duration of the seizure
Observe the details

Call for help if:
Hurt (injury is necessary for medical attention)
Exclusive (their first seizure ever)
Longer than five minutes
Plural (they have more than one seizure; seizures repeat without full recovery)

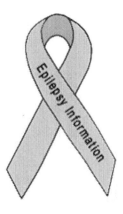

Treatment Options

Epilepsy is a battle in itself, yet alone finding the right treatment. Unfortunately, not everyone will reach his or her goal of seizure free living, at least not with the first try or type of treatment. The beauty is there are many options for treatments and maybe even cures. Even if you have struggled with epilepsy your entire life with little to no seizure control, it does not mean you should quit trying. Research continues to bring new options to the table giving you a fresh chance at living your life seizure free!

Antiepileptic Medications

Medication is the first line of defense against seizure activity. Treatment through medication is a tricky balancing act. You need enough medication to stop the seizures. However, too much medication can cause negative side effects. The key is to find a happy medium. Before you get started, you need to accept there is no "rhyme or reason." When it comes to finding the right medication at the right dose, it is a guessing game. You may need to try a few different medications, mix of medications, and dosing adjustments. All the "fine tuning" can take a few months.

There is a large range of medications on the market with more to come. See: *Medications and Possible Side Effects*

Even if you're feeling well, talk to your doctor about adjusting your medication if you have:

- Good control but not complete control
- Strong undesirable side effects

It may take several months before the best medication(s) and dosage(s) are determined for you. During this adjustment period, you will be carefully monitored through frequent blood tests to measure blood levels as well as your response to the medication. It is very important to keep your follow-up appointments as well as the laboratory to minimize the risk for serious side effects and prevent complications.

DIETARY TREATMENT

Sometimes seizures are intractable and continue despite medication, even with aggressive medication treatment. As children's precious little brains are being attacked by seizures, they can be gaining ground over possibly controlling them with a special diet! However, it's important to note, therapeutic diets are just as serious as medication and need to be monitored. No diet to treat epilepsy should be done without a neurologist's and dietitian's involvement.

Ketogenic Diet

Like other therapies for epilepsy, it has side effects that must be watched for. Take caution in attempting to put your child on the diet without their doctor's care. *It is not a "do-it-yourself" diet.* It is a very serious form of treatment. In fact, the diet is usually started in the hospital. It's usually not feasible in older children or adults.

General candidates are children in the range of one to twelve years of age in whom medication has not helped. Studies have shown the diet may be of use with adults that do not benefit from medication as well. If effective after the two month trial period, the diet typically continues for two years. It involves calculations but is not hard to do. A dietitian will guide and help you with menus. However, if you want the best possible results you will need to understand how the diet works intensely so you can do some "fine tuning" as needed.

Basic materials necessary:
- Calculator
- Electronic weight scales (accurate to one gram)
- Food tables
- Ketodiastix (urine testing strips)
- Measuring cups
- Sugar free toothpaste
- Vitamin supplements

There is absolutely **no** *room for "cheating" on this diet.* You must stick to the diet all the time because the slightest deviation from the diet can actually *cause* seizures. Since the steadfastness of the diet is so demanded, your child must take meals and or snacks to school and social occasions. Their teacher and other school officials must know the seriousness of your child sticking to the diet. It may seem overwhelming when you first start the diet however, like everything else it gets easier with time as it starts to feel natural.

Process:
- Your child will be hospitalized.
- A registered dietician will monitor them.
- Their medications will initially remain unchanged.
- They'll fast for approximately one to two days.
- The diet will start on the second or third day.
- Over several months to a year, the diet will be "tweaked" accordingly.
- They'll maintain on the diet for two years.
- After two years, they'll be weaned off.

Possible side effects:
- Nausea
- Vomiting
- Diarrhea
- Constipation

- Dehydration
- Loss of energy (first few days)
- Bone fractures
- High cholesterol levels
- Irritability
- Slowed growth, weight gain or loss (generally "catch up" after diet is ended)
- Malnutrition (if supplements are neglected)

Less common and potentially more serious side effects include:
- Susceptibility to infections
- Anemia
- High cholesterol
- Low protein
- Kidney stones
- Thinning of the bones

The nutritional program consists of two phases, healing and maintenance. The diet promotes eating a lot of lean meat, fish, eggs, green leafy and other non-starchy veggies, fruit in moderation, unrefined grains in moderation, nuts, seeds, and all the "good" fats and proteins your body needs such as avocados, flaxseed oil, butter, mayonnaise, and olive oil.

Benefits:
- Lower blood pressure
- Improved digestion
- During diet, possible reduction of a.e.d.s
- 50% patients have less seizure activity
- 15% patients become seizure free
- Improved alertness
- Improved sleep
- Most improvements in seizure control that result from the diet will be permanent.

Disadvantages:
- Because of highly restrictive guidelines, it's tempting to "stray."
- Having to remain in ketosis, can make it difficult to find appropriate foods at social functions, school, and restaurants.
- Can be detrimental in long-term health.

Risks:
- Lower blood pressure
- Dehydration
- Constipation
- Vomiting
- Thinning bones
- May cause injury to brain cells that help control body weight.
- High cholesterol level
- Kidney stones
- Behavioral changes
- Slower growth rates

Example of typical daily menu:

Breakfast:
- Scrambled eggs
- Nitrate-free sausages
- 2/3 cup oatmeal with butter and cream
- Sliced tomatoes

Snack:
- String cheese

Lunch:
- Salad (salad greens, chicken, hard boiled egg, nitrate-free bacon, blue cheese, tomatoes, olive oil, and vinegar dressing)
- Small apple

Dinner:
- Roast pork loin
- 1/3 cup brown rice with butter
- Asparagus with butter
- Salad greens with cucumbers and tomatoes
- Olive oil and vinegar dressing

Typical meals for the diet may include small amounts of fruits and vegetables, which contain carbohydrates, large servings of fatty foods such as eggs, butter, and heavy cream; and a small portion of protein-rich meat or fish. For recipes, meal ideas, and much more go to charliefoundation.org

Low Glycemic Index Treatment (L.G.I.T.)

Attempts to reproduce the positive effects of the ketogenic diet. The glycemic index is the measurement of a particular food's effect on blood-sugar levels. High glycemic index foods contain simple sugars such as table sugar, which quickly raise your blood sugar after eating. Many grains have a low glycemic index because they affect blood-sugar levels slower than high glycemic index foods. Counting carbohydrates and rough portion control is usually sufficient for the diet to have a seizure-reducing effect.

Basic materials necessary:
- Multivitamins
- Calcium
- Minerals

Process:
- You will start as an outpatient.
- You won't need to weigh your food.
- A registered dietician will monitor you.

Possible side effects:
- Changes in blood chemistry
- Constipation
- Weight loss

Benefits:
- Hospitalization is not necessary.
- Reduces seizures (sometimes by more than 90%).
- Easier to follow than ketogenic diet.
- Offers wider range of food than ketogenic diet.
- Appropriate food for diet can be ordered in cafeterias and restaurants.
- If successful in controlling seizures, it may be continued for several years.

Differences from ketogenic diet:

- Allows for a broader range of food types.
- Does not require weighing.
- Carbohydrate intake is less restricted.
- Allows for approximately four times as many grams of carbohydrates (if they come from foods with low glycemic index).

Disadvantages:

- Diet needs commitment to lifestyle participation in order to maintain seizure control.

Risks:

- Can increase cholesterol
- Heart disease
- Malnutrition (if supplements are neglected)
- Reduced growth in children
- Reduced bone mass

Example of typical daily menu:

Breakfast:
- Fruit with yogurt smoothie

Lunch:
- Grilled ham with Swiss cheese on rye bread
- Fruit

Dinner:
- Baked chicken breast
- Vegetables with lentil

Modified Atkins Diet

Modification of the ketogenic diet. The foods are similar (high in fat and low in carbohydrates). However, there are key differences between the two. Children can eat more foods, and can "cheat" with some breads and cake products as long as the total carbohydrates per day remain below the set amount prescribed by the dietician.

Even so, it's still a hard diet. Teens are more likely to be considered for this diet due to flexibility. Like the ketogenic diet, if the child's seizure free for a two year period, the diet can stop successfully.

Basic materials necessary:
- Multivitamins
- Calcium
- Minerals
- Urine ketone strips

Process:
- You will start the diet as an outpatient.
- For the first month, you'll be allowed ten grams of carbohydrates daily or 15 – 20 (if ten is too restrictive).
- You'll be monitored by a registered dietician.
- You're diet will be individualized.
- Multivitamin, mineral, and calcium supplements are required.
- Goals are provided based on your current diet intake and growth history.
- Your carbohydrate intake is restricted to ensure the diet meets caloric needs.
- You'll eat carbohydrates, fats, and proteins together.
- You'll have occasional blood work.
- Your medication may be reduced over time.

Possible side effects:
- Constipation
- Kidney stones
- Slow growth
- Changes in blood chemistry
- Feeling of hunger (even if calories are not reduced)
- Low bone density
- Weight loss

Benefits:
- Less restrictive than traditional ketogenic diet.
- No measuring or weighing foods.
- Shorter "hangover" time after seizures.

- Healthy bowel function.
- Changes can be made, if necessary.
- Wider range of foods and fewer side effects than traditional ketogenic diet.
- Calories are not restricted.
- Reduction in medication.
- Improves clarity of thought and ability to make decisions.
- Lowers risk of heart disease, diabetes, and cancer.

Differences from ketogenic diet:
- No weighing and measuring foods.
- No restriction of fluids or calories.
- Fats are strongly encouraged.
- No restrictions on proteins.
- You do not have to follow specific meal plans.
- Typical carbohydrate intake is twenty grams.
- Hospitalization is not required.
- Fasting is not necessary.
- Foods can be eaten more freely in restaurants and outside the home.

Disadvantages:
- Appropriate for orally fed patients only.
- Desired result is less than ketogenic diet.

Risks:
- *Weight loss*
- Possibility of elevated bad cholesterol
- Dehydration (if you lose the desire to drink)
- Malnutrition (if supplements are neglected)

Example of typical daily menu:

Breakfast:
- Omelet with cheese
- Cream
- Butter
- Tomato

Lunch:
- Cream of chicken soup with vegetable of choice

Dinner:
- Sausage
- Parsnip chips
- Mushrooms
- Raspberry cream yogurt

SURGERY

There are two kinds of epilepsy surgery, curative and palliative. Curative attempts to stop the seizures, and palliative restricts the spread of the seizures. Most patients with epilepsy do not require surgery. However, if medications are ineffective after a certain period, surgery can be an appropriate option for treatment for some types of epilepsy. If there's no control over seizures with medication, you may be a candidate for surgery. However, surgery is an individual decision and not all patients are candidates.

Evaluation Prior to Surgery Once it has been determined, that the seizures relate to epilepsy and you have not improved after aggressive medication therapy, and surgery is the next step, a range of tests will be the next step! The testing will help locate the seizure focus and provide the surgeon with valuable information about your brain. The exact tests depend on the type of epilepsy and type of surgery planned.

Probable tests prior to surgery:
- E.E.G. (external)
- E.E.G. (subdural and depth electrodes)
- Video E.E.G.
- M.R.I.
- F.M.R.I.
- P.E.T.
- S.P.E.C.T.
- Complete physical

- Extensive medical history (review of seizure type, frequency, and seizure duration)
- Neuropsychological testing
- Psychiatric evaluation
- Visual field evaluation
- Wada

Consideration for surgery may include:
- Intractable seizures.
- Partial seizures that always start in one area of your brain (localized seizure focus).
- Seizure discharge that spreads to the whole brain (secondary generalization).
- Seizures caused by a lesion such as scar tissue, a brain tumor, or AVM (birth defect).
- Seizures significantly affecting your quality of life.
- Severe side effects to the medications.

Palliative Surgery

Palliative procedures are necessary when a specific area of the brain or seizure focus cannot be determined. These procedures do not remove any area of the brain. Instead, they prevent the spread of seizures or reduce their frequency and/or severity.

Corpus Callosotomy

Procedure that severs the membrane which divides the right and left cerebral hemispheres that interfere with the electrical process of the seizure. It's usually necessary to do in two stages unless improvement is significant after the first. The first stage of surgery involves dividing the front two thirds of the corpus callosum leaving the rest intact. The second stage is to divide the remaining portion. The corpus callosotomy does not usually stop the patient from having seizures. It may actually increase the frequency of certain kinds of localized seizures. This surgery is not necessary with hope of curing seizures, but rather with hope of helping to reduce their severity.

Corpus callosotomy is more commonly performed on children when:
- There is no single focus.
- The focus is inoperable.
- The seizures are generalized.
- A resection of a localized focus would cause a pronounced neurological deficit.

Procedure is often done in stages:
- Your child will be placed asleep under general anesthesia.
- Their head will be shaved.
- An incision will be made to open and remove a portion of their skull.
- The two hemispheres will be sectioned.

  ► For a partial callosotomy the anterior two-thirds of the brain are sectioned.

  ► If necessary, a complete callosotomy (additional surgery from anterior section) in the posterior one- third is also sectioned.

- After sectioning, the dura is closed.
- The skull portion will be replaced and stitched with non magnetic wire, staples, and/or titanium plates.
- Their scalp will be stitched together.
- Their head will be wrapped with gauze.
- *Surgery typically takes up to six hours.*

Gamma knife is an alternative approach. See: *Glossary*

After procedure:
- Your child will be taken to I.C.U. until they are medically stable enough to go to another nursing unit.
- While they're in I.C.U., they will be monitored closely *(blood pressure, pulse, respirations, temperature, and pain control)*.
- Inpatient or outpatient rehabilitation may be necessary to optimize their functioning.
- They will be evaluated over the next several months, (to check effectiveness of the first surgery and evaluate if the second surgery is necessary).

- Several weeks of convalescence at home are required before your child can resume normal activities.
- *They may return to school in 6 – 8 weeks.*

Benefits:
- Seizure frequency is reduced by an average of 70% – 80% after a partial, 80% – 90% after a complete.
- Intractable drop attacks (tonic and atonic seizures), tonic–clonic, absence, and frontal lobe complex partial seizures respond well.
- Reduction or discontinuation of medication.
- Reduced seizure frequency (50% or more patients).
- Significantly reduced seizure severity.
- Some patients become seizure free.
- Atonic seizures are eliminated (70%).

Disadvantage:
- Inpatient or outpatient therapy may be necessary.
- May need two surgeries.

Risks:
- Swelling
- Infection
- Behavioral changes
- Decreased spontaneity of speech
- Decreased use of non-dominant hand
- Difficulty with right/left confusion (can improve with speech and physical therapy)
- Hemorrhage (less than 1%)
- Mutism (unable to speak)
- Subtle deficits (connecting words with images)
- Temporary or permanent limitations of speech
- Temporary or permanent limitations of movement of certain body parts.

Although corpus callosotomy has been performed since 1940 to treat severe medically intractable seizures, there remains controversy as to when, or even if, the surgery should be performed.

Deep Brain Stimulator (D.B.S.)

A surgically implanted device, similar to a cardiac pacemaker, originally designed to control symptoms of Parkinson's disease. It delivers continuous electrical stimulation to targeted areas in your brain. The intention of the DBS is to provide treatment for patients whose seizures do not respond to anti epileptic medication therapy. The stimulator targets the thalamus which is the part of the brain that produces most epileptic seizures. Some studies revealed more than half the patients treated during the trials experienced a reduction of epileptic seizures by at least fifty percent.

Surgery:
- You will be placed asleep under general anesthesia.
- A lightweight frame will be placed on your skull.
- A series of brain scans will determine exact positioning of the leads.
- Burr holes are drilled on either side of the skull.
- The electrodes go through the skull to the target area.
- When the electrodes are placed, the holes are closed.
- The other end of the DBS leads (not containing electrodes) are connected individually to two extension cables.
- The extension cables are tunneled under the skin behind the ear, to the chest wall on the same side of the neck.
- They are both connected to the stimulator, which is then put into a small "pocket" under the skin.
- Another scan is performed to assure the electrodes are positioned correctly.
- All the wounds are closed and dressed.
- The doctor uses radio waves to program the implanted device. This part of the process is neither painful nor invasive.
- The doctor can adjust many variables, including which electrodes are selected to ensure the best effect is achieved.
- *The length of the operation usually lasts between 3 – 6 hours.*

After surgery:
- The stimulator may be programmed either immediately or within a few days.
- *The recovery period usually lasts between 3 – 5 days.*

Benefits:
- Adjustable
- Brain remains intact
- Removable
- Reduced seizures
- *Reduced medication*

Disadvantages:
- The presence of a foreign object in the body may increase the risk of infection.
- Repeat surgery every 3 – 5 years in order to replace the battery.
- Uncomfortable sensations that may occur during stimulation.

Risks:
- Stroke (1 – 3%)
- Intracranial hemorrhage.
- Headaches.
- Erosion of the plastic cable or device through the skin.
- The plastic cap that anchors the deep brain stimulation wire to the skull can break.
- Numbness of the face, arm, hand or leg.
- Change in mood.
- Thinking problems.
- Feeling of light headedness.
- The stimulator can be adjusted to treat side effects.

M.S.T.
(Multiple Subpial Transection)

Procedure is used to help control seizures that begin in areas of the brain that cannot be safely removed. The surgeon makes a series of shallow cuts (transections) in the brain tissue. These cuts interrupt the movement of seizure impulses but do not disturb normal brain activity, leaving the person's abilities intact. This technique may be used alone or in combination with a lobectomy. It has been proposed as an *appropriate treatment for Landau-Kleffner syndrome.*

Surgery:

- You will be asleep under general anesthesia.
- An incision will be made in your scalp.
- A piece of your skull will be removed.
- A section of the dura is pulled back.
- A series of parallel, shallow cuts are made in the gray matter.
- The dura is fixed back into place.
- The skull portion will be replaced and stitched with non magnetic wire, staples, and/or titanium plates.
- Your scalp will be closed with stitches.
- Your head will be wrapped with gauze.

After surgery:

- You'll go to I.C.U. for 24 – 48 hours.
- In 3 – 4 days or until medically stable enough, you'll go to another nursing unit.
- *You may return to your normal activities, including work or school in 6 – 8 weeks.*
- You will continue to take anti-seizure medication.
- Once seizure control is established, medications may be reduced or eliminated.

Benefits:

- 70% of patients experience satisfactory improvement in seizure control.
- Intended to be used in cases where lesions are "unresectable," due to areas of the brain that will affect the memory, speech, memory, and sensory functions.
- Children with LKS or other forms of epilepsy uncontrolled by medication may have improved or psychosocial functioning.

Disadvantages:

- Invasive
- Inpatient care

Risks:

- Infection
- Bleeding

- Swelling in the brain
- Damage to healthy brain tissue

R.N.S.
(Responsive Neurostimulator)

The RNS system is the first closed-loop responsive brain stimulation system used to treat intractable partial onset seizures. It's a programmable, battery powered, microprocessor-controlled device that delivers a short train of electrical pulses to the brain through implanted leads. It continuously monitors the brain's electrical activity through electrodes which detects abnormal activity.

The system includes implantable and external products. The implantable components include the stimulator and the leads. The external products include the programmer, a laptop computer with software that has a wand, and transmitter enabling communication with the implanted device. Doctors use the programmer to noninvasively program the detection and stimulation of the device. Additional features of the programmer include the ability to view the patient's brain electrical activity (electrocorticogram or ECoG) in real-time and the ability to upload the patient's ECoGs that have been stored in the RNS.

The device trials started in April 2006. On December 7, 2009, NeuroPace announced the results from the trial. On February 25, 2013, the FDA Neurological Devices panel voted unanimously (11 – 0) that the clinical benefits far outweigh the risks. The system is an investigational device limited by the United States for investigational purposes. It will be available after the study commitments have been satisfied and approved. If you would like to follow the progression regarding this system, go to Neuropace.com

Surgery:
- You will be asleep under general anesthesia.
- An incision will be made to open and remove a portion of your skull.
- The device is implanted in the skull connected to one to two leads containing electrodes.

- The electrodes are placed inside or rest on the brain surface at the seizure focus.
- The skull portion will be replaced and stitched with non magnetic wire, staples, and/or titanium plates.
- Your scalp will be closed with stitches.
- Your head will be wrapped with gauze.
- *Hospitalization typically lasts up to four days.*

After surgery:

- The doctor will program the detection and stimulation of the R.N.S. to customize the therapy for your specific needs.
- The device will deliver brief mild stimulation in order to suppress the seizure *before* the symptoms occur.
- You will be able to return to your normal activities, including work or school, in 6 – 8 weeks.
- The hair over the incision will grow back and hide the surgical scar.
- Most patients will need to continue taking anti-seizure medication for two or more years after surgery. Once seizure control is established, medications may be reduced or eliminated.

Benefits:

- Battery replacement procedures can be performed on an outpatient basis.
- The device can be programmed noninvasively.
- May provide a safe and effective treatment.
- Safe for patients with partial onset and generalized tonic-clonic seizures.
- Seizure frequency reduced up to 53% (according to a two year trial study).
- Ability to view the patient's brain electrical activity in real time.
- Uploads the EcoG's that have been stored in the device.

Disadvantage:

- Replacement of batteries is required every two years along with replacement of the device.

Risks:

- Infection
- Bleeding
- Changes in personality or mental abilities

V.N.S.
(Vagus Nerve Stimulator)

Reduces severity of seizures through electrical stimulation of the vagus nerve. The nerve begins at the brain stem and passes through the cranial cavity past the jugular, to the throat, larynx, lungs, heart, esophagus, stomach, and abdomen.

The VNS consists of a titanium-encased generator, the size of a pocket watch. It receives its power from a lithium battery, with a battery life of six to eight years. It consists of a lead system with electrodes, and an anchor tether to secure leads to the vagus nerve. Implantation of the VNS is usually done as an outpatient procedure. It appears to be efficient enough for seizures that do not respond well to medications alone but is commonly used with the assistance of medication. The degree of effectiveness is approximately the same as newly marketed medications. Patients of any age, including infants, may be candidates for surgery if they meet other criteria.

Surgery:
- You will be sound asleep under general anesthesia.
- An incision is made in your upper left chest.
- The generator is implanted into a little "pouch" on the left chest under the clavicle (collar bone).
- A second incision is made in the neck, so the surgeon can access the vagus nerve.
- The surgeon then wraps the leads around the left branch of the vagus nerve, and connects the electrodes to the generator.
- *The surgery lasts approximately two hours.*

The left vagus nerve is stimulated rather than the right because the right plays a role in cardiac function. Stimulating the right nerve could have negative cardiac effects.

After surgery:
- Battery powered device will be programmed from outside of your body by your doctor.

Benefits:
- Stimulation can be adjusted by you with a hand held magnet.

- Sends electric impulses to the vagus nerve at *regular* intervals.
- No major surgery is necessary.
- Your brain is not disturbed.

In studies:
- After three months, seizures decreased by 1/3.
- After 12 months, seizures decreased by 1/2.
- Effective in some children.
- Improved learning, independence, and mood in some children.

Disadvantages:
- There will be a slight bulge where the device is implanted.
- *You'll have small* scars on your neck where the wire leads were placed and the device was implanted.
- It doesn't replace medication.
- May cause increased hyperactivity in children.
- It's not a cure.
- It doesn't work for everyone.

Risks:
- Infection
- Swallowing difficulty
- Sleep apnea
- Coughing
- Scratchy, sore throat
- Hoarseness or slight voice changes
- Overall, the treatment is considered safe.

Research has shown it may reduce seizures in about 30 – 40% of patients. For more information contact: Cyberonics 888-VNS-STIM or vnstherapy.com

Curative Surgery

Before consideration of curative surgery, an evaluation is performed to ensure the operation will remove seizure activity as well as not cause damage to essential functions such as speech, vision, and memory. Eligibility for surgery is determined jointly by your epileptologist, neuroradiologist, neurosurgeon, neuropsychologist, and social worker. The decision to have the surgery is made jointly by you and your epileptologist after carefully reviewing the benefits and risks.

During surgery, the area of the brain that triggers the seizures (usually a portion of a lobe) is removed. After surgery, some patients will be completely free of seizures. Others will have better control over the seizures. Some patients may need additional surgery.

When you discover surgery is an option, be sure to review the risks and benefits with your doctor. Do not rely on the internet. You will get conflicting information! Your epileptologist and neurosurgeon is the source you should trust most to review all the risks and benefits.

Hemispherectomy

The candidate for a hemispherectomy has epilepsy with intractable seizures, numerous of ill-defined focal points yet localized to one hemisphere. Such patients may have one or a wide variety of disorders that have caused seizures, including:

- Hemimegalencephaly
- Neonatal brain injury
- Rasmussen syndrome
- Sturge-Weber syndrome

Functional Hemispherectomy

Involves disconnection of one side of the brain from the other, and removal of almost an entire half of the brain (hemisphere) with some tissue left in place.

This surgery is almost exclusively performed on children who:
- Have severely damaged hemispheres.
- Are typically partially paralyzed on the side of the body opposite of the diseased hemisphere.
- Usually have intractable seizures.
- Have weakness on one side of the body.
- Sometimes have a smaller hand.

Prior to both hemispherectomies:

- You will be placed asleep under general anesthesia.
- Your head will be shaved.
- A portion of your skull will be removed.
- A portion of the temporal lobe will be removed.
- A corpus callosotomy is performed.
- Frontal and occipital lobes are disconnected.
- Underlying tissues are stitched.
- The skull portion will be replaced and stitched with non magnetic wire, staples, and/or titanium plates.
- Your scalp will be closed with stitches.
- Your head will be wrapped with gauze.

Immediately after the operation, you may be on a mechanical ventilator for up to 24 hours. You will remain in the hospital for at least one week for physical and occupational therapy to improve strength and motor function.

Benefits:

- Cognitive functioning, attention span, and behavior may improve.
- Able to walk with some rehabilitation.
- Seizures are eliminated in 70 – 85% of patients.
- Seizures are reduced by 80%.
- Medications may be slowly tapered off for some patients after a seizure-free period of one year.
- Some improvement in intellectual function may occur.

Disadvantages:

- Invasive
- Two surgeries may be necessary

Side effects:

- Scalp numbness
- Nausea
- Muscle weakness on the affected side of body
- Puffy eyes
- Feeling tired or depressed

- Difficulty speaking, remembering, or finding words
- Headaches

Risks:
- Limited functioning
- Hemisphere damage
- Loss of movement or sensation on the opposite side of the body
- Loss of peripheral vision
- Hemorrhage
- Hydrocephalus
- Infection
- Brain swelling
- Delayed development
- Persistent seizures
- Death (1 – 2%)

Lobectomies

If it comes time to decide whether or not to have surgery, don't allow the fear of pain stop you! Yes, it'll hurt badly. But all surgeries do. Ask yourself what's worse, years or even a lifetime of seizures or a few days of a really bad headache! I chose the headache, and trust me it was well worth it!

Frontal Lobectomy

The frontal lobectomy is the second most common type of epilepsy surgery. However, the success rates are not as good as those for temporal lobectomy. Approximately 30% – 50% of patients have better seizure control. Behavioral changes in mood, motivation, organization, and personality are more common with this procedure.

Parietal and Occipital Lobectomies

These types of lobectomies are uncommon. Locating a seizure focus in one of these lobes is more difficult, and usually requires subdural electrodes. The risks of surgery in the parietal or occipital lobes depend on the area removed.

Temporal Lobectomy

The most common type of epilepsy surgery for people with temporal lobe epilepsy. The risks of surgery are relatively low. After surgery as the brain heals, seizures may flare up for one to two months. However, seizure activity during the postoperative months does not mean the operation was unsuccessful. In fact, 75% of epilepsy surgeries are successful! You may be able to go off all medications possibly within a year's time after surgery.

Surgery is not usually a means of a cure. You may still have occasional simple partial auras or rarely breakthrough seizures. Twenty-five percent of patients do not respond favorably to seizure surgery, usually due to the fact the seizures were multi-focal or all of the focus area could not be removed.

Surgery:
- The surgery begins after you are positioned and placed asleep under general anesthesia.
- A patch of your hair is shaved over the temple area. (It's not necessary to shave your entire head).
- Your skin is cut into a c-shaped partial circle above your ear.
- Several nickel-sized holes are drilled in a circular pattern.
- A bone-saw cuts between the holes to remove a circle of bone approximately the circumference of a small coffee cup rim.
- The dura mater (membrane over the brain), is cut open exposing the temporal lobe.
- Portions of the temporal lobe are removed by suction because the brain has a firm 'pudding-like' consistency. The usual amount removed ranges between the size of a golf ball and a small lemon. (about half the volume of the temporal lobe)
- The skull portion will be replaced and stitched with non magnetic wire, staples, and/or titanium plates.
- Your scalp will be closed with stitches.
- Your head will be wrapped with gauze.
- *The operation itself usually takes about two to three hours.*
- *You will be ideally in the operating room* and *recovery room combined for 4 – 8 hours.*

After surgery:

- Pain or itching around the scar (especially as it heals).
- You will be disoriented for a day.
- You'll experience migraine-like persistent headaches for one to two weeks.
- You may have a sore throat from the breathing tube during surgery.
- Swelling and bruising of the forehead and eye on the side of surgery is likely. (The swelling increases to a peak 2 – 4 days after surgery).
- *You'll spend at least two days in I.C.U.*
- After day three, you may be able to sit in a chair, walk with assistance, and eat.
- Until you're able to eat, pain medication will be given through IV.
- If no complications occur, you'll be discharged within three to six days.
- You'll notice skull indentations and bumps from the wire and/or plates.
- Numbness at the surgical site.
- Plan on resting at home with assistance for at least a week.
- You should not return to work or perform any heavy activities for at least one month.

Benefits:

- Non magnetic wire *will calcify to reseal the bone and never needs removed*.
- Plates if used *rarely* need replaced.
- The portion of brain removed will fill with the fluid surrounding the brain and never grows back.
- Surgery is successful about 75%.
- Patients may be able to reduce or stop all medications one year after surgery.

Disadvantages:

- Invasive.
- Inpatient care.
- Surgery is not usually the means of a cure but better control over seizures.

Less serious, more common risks:

- Deterioration of word-finding ability (a few months after surgery).
- Drooping of forehead or eyelid on the surgical side.
- Minor loss of upper peripheral vision on the opposite side of the surgery.
- Short-lived depression.
- Memory loss.

Severe/rare Risks:

- Death (0.1 – 0.5%)
- Hemorrhage 2%
- Infection
- Memory ability deterioration
- Partial paralysis
- Partial vision loss
- Personality change
- Psychiatric deterioration
- Reading difficulties
- Severe depression
- Severe speech problems
- Stroke

A surgically produced scar <u>rarely</u> leads to seizures because it's closed in reverse order to the opening.

If you have exhausted all your options for treatment with little or no seizure control, do not give up hope! Scientists have not quit searching for new medications, devices, surgeries, and of course a cure. Since the medical world will never give up, you shouldn't either because it's not over yet.

Keep your eyes open for new treatments! Keep asking your doctor and searching the web. Never tire! The next treatment might be the right one for you!

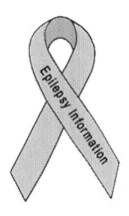

Epilepsy Information

Medications
and Possible Side Effects

(Generics are in parentheses)

Antiepileptic medications can cause unwanted side effects in some people. The majority of the time the effects are mild and short lasting. Finding the correct medication(s) and dosage amounts can be a tedious time to go through. However, just because side effects exist does not mean you will experience them. Inform your doctor as soon as possible if any side effects develop or change in intensity. Only your doctor can determine if it is safe for you to continue, discontinue or change your medication. Do not make any medical decisions based on the following information.

If the information provided in this chapter causes you concern, it's in your best interest to discuss it with your doctor and/or their nurse. They can go over the symptoms in which they see more often or not at all! Serious side effects are rare. Do not hinder yourself from trying a medication due to the possible side effects. In addition, do not stop taking your medication unless your doctor instructs you to do so. Please remember, your risk of harm from a seizure is far greater than the risk of side effects from medication.

If insurance and/or finances are an issue and you cannot afford your medication. See: *Patient Assistance Programs and Discount Prescripton Cards*

Generic vs. Brand Name

There is reason to believe there is a big enough discrepancy between brand name and generic medication that can be incompatible with seizure control. Some people's seizure activity is so vulnerable that a minute change from brand name to generic or vice versa can cause preventable seizure activity. Therefore, continuing with either generic or brand name appears to be the best method now until research offers more information. In other words, if the brand name medication successfully controls the seizures continue using it! On the other hand, if generic medications work keep using them! Generics get a bad name but are not automatically the problem. It is the switching around that appears to be the problem.

However, since there is no clinical evidence to confirm there is a dilemma amongst epilepsy patients and generic medication, both pharmacies and insurance companies can change your medications without foreknowledge or authorization. Nevertheless you can take charge of the situation. If the brand name proves to be successful, have your doctor write, 'brand name medically necessary' on *every* prescription. And if the generic is successful, have your doctor write 'generic name medically necessary' on *every* prescription. You need to include the manufacturer's name on every prescription since many companies make generics for the same medication! (Manufacturer names can be found on the prescription bottle). This will prevent flip-flopping with your medication.

Three types of side effects:

The information in this chapter may cause you to be alarmed but remember the benefits from AEDs far outweigh the risks in almost every case of possible side effects. The more serious side effects are very uncommon. Most undesirable side effects are short lasting and reversible. In rare cases however, medication can actually worsen seizures.

Idiosyncratic are rare and unpredictable reactions, which are not dose-related. They most often include, low blood cell counts, liver problems, and skin rashes.

Unique are unshared by other drugs in the same class. For example, medication #1 can cause the gums to swell and medication #2 can cause hair loss. Ask your doctor about unique side effects before taking the medication.

Common or predictable occur with any antiepileptic medication because they affect the central nervous system and are dose-related, generic, and nonspecific. The side effects include blurry or double vision, fatigue, sleepiness, unsteadiness, and upset stomach.

Ways to distinguish side effects:
- Usually start 30 minutes to two hours after the medication is taken.
- Last more than 15 minutes.
- Appear shortly after a new medication is started.
- Appear shortly after a recently increased dosage.

Pay close attention to see if the symptoms occur when taken:
- Close together
- On an empty stomach
- With food
- With small amounts of liquid

The following medications cause bone loss:
- Tegretol, Carbatrol (Carbamazepine)
- Dilantin (Phenytek)
- Phenobarbital (Phenytoin)
- Primidone (Mysoline)
- Topamax (Topiramate)
- Depakote (Valproate)

You should discuss taking calcium with your doctor to ensure you are taking the proper dosage. The typical range is 1200 – 1800 mg. with vitamin D daily at 600 mg. intervals. *You can only absorb 600 mg. at a time.*

It is in your best interest to avoid driving, operating dangerous machinery or participating in activities that requires full mental alertness until you are certain the medication does not have a debilitating effect. If you experience a serious side effect, you and/or your doctor may send a report to the Food and Drug Administration (FDA). Go Med Watch Adverse Event reporting program at fda.gov/medwatch or call (800) 332-1088.

Steps to report serious side effects online:

- Print FDA 3500 Voluntary report.
- Fill out the form with specific details.
- Give it to your doctor so they can send it in.

AEDs determination for legalization of a new medication goes by the following traits:

- Frequency
- Medical history
- Overall health
- Area of the brain affected
- Age
- Possible side affects
- Severity
- Seizure type (focal, partial vs. generalized, etc.)

An accurate diagnosis of the type of epilepsy is critical in choosing the best treatment for you. As you can see in the following lists, there are many medications currently used to treat epilepsy. These medications control specific types of seizures, so don't be alarmed if you aren't gaining control over seizures, and your doctor will not try every medication on the market! It will not help to try a medication just because it exists. However, people who have more than one type of seizure may have to take more than one medication. Actually, it's common for people with one type of seizure to take more than one medication. Just like anything else in life, you do whatever it takes to get the result you desire.

Every new medication must go through a trial period in which patients volunteer to try the medications to see the outcome of symptoms, improvement, and side effects. If more than one person suffers from the same effect, it must be reported and listed as a possible side effect. Therefore, some side effects may have been experienced just a couple times! Therefore, the majority of the side effects listed are uncommon or unlikely. However, the true picture of product safety actually evolves over months or even years that make up its lifetime in the marketplace.

The clinical trials that help determine product safety are conducted on small groups of patients. Which means a range from a few hundred to several thousand problems can remain hidden or show up at all. They may only be revealed after thousands of people or more use the product! In a roundabout way it means, if the drug is new on the market, you are taking part in the trial!

There are many issues to work through with new medications. For instance, clinical trials cannot assess the effects of every new medication in combination with other approved medications. Therefore, it is possible that a patient could have a serious reaction from a new medication when taken with another medication in a combination that was not tested in a trial. However, if you try a medication, which is new on the market and you experience a serious side effect, which is not recorded, you have the responsibility to report it. The same goes for medications that have been on the market for years.

Allergic reactions are usually within the first six months and are infrequent but do occur. A rash is the most common allergic reaction.

Unpredictable side effects, not related to the dosage or medication blood level, can include:
- Inflammation or failure of the liver, kidney, or bone marrow
- Rash
- Reduction in platelet count
- Reduction in white blood cells

If overdose is suspected, contact the American Association of Poison Control Centers (800) 222-1222 or go to your nearest emergency room immediately.

Tell your doctor if any of the symptoms listed are severe and/or do not go away.

Ativan (Lorazepam)
- Dizziness
- Weakness
- Unsteadiness
- Fatigue
- Memory loss
- Confusion
- Vertigo
- Blurred vision
- Nausea
- Slurred speech
- Headaches

Banzel (Refinamide)
- Depression
- Anxiety
- Suicidal thoughts
- Aggression
- Rash
- Hives
- Itching
- Unexplained swelling
- Wheezing
- Difficulty breathing or swallowing

Carbatrol (Carbamazepine)
- Anxiety
- Back pain
- Constipation
- Drowsiness
- Diarrhea
- Dizziness
- Dry mouth
- Headache
- Heartburn
- Memory problems

- Unsteadiness
- Upset stomach
- Vomiting
- Insomnia
- Nervousness
- Headache

Comfyde (Carisbamate)
- Dizziness
- Headache
- Nausea
- Sleepy

Depakene (Valproic acid)
- Abnormal thinking
- Agitation
- Back pain
- Changes in appetite
- Dizziness
- Blurred or double vision
- Constipation
- Diarrhea
- Hair loss
- Drowsiness
- Headache
- Uncontrollable shaking of a body part
- Heartburn
- Mood swings
- Runny or stuffy nose
- Memory loss
- Ringing in the ears
- Weight changes
- Loss of coordination
- Sore throat
- Uncontrollable movements of the eyes

Depakote (Divalproex sodium, Valproic acid)
- Back pain
- Blurred or double vision

- Constipation
- Dizziness
- Changes in appetite
- Agitation
- Hair loss
- Abnormal thinking
- Diarrhea
- Drowsiness
- Headache
- Heartburn
- Loss of coordination
- Uncontrollable shaking of a part of the body
- Mood swings
- Ringing in the ears
- Sore throat
- Memory loss
- Runny or stuffy nose
- Uncontrollable movements of the eyes
- Weight changes

Diamox (Acetazolamide)
- Upset stomach
- Vomiting
- Loss of appetite
- Numbness and tingling
- Drowsiness

Diastat (Diazepam)
- Diarrhea
- Flushing
- Headache
- Drowsiness
- Pain
- Problems falling asleep or staying asleep
- Dizziness
- Abnormal "high" mood
- Lack of coordination
- Stomach pain
- Nervousness

- Runny nose
- Unsteadiness

Dilantin (Phenytoin)
- Blurred or double vision
- Headache
- Difficulty swallowing
- Drowsiness
- Insomnia
- Loss of taste and appetite
- Nervousness
- Mental confusion
- Constipation
- Muscle twitching
- Redness, irritation, bleeding, and swelling of the gums
- Weight loss
- Stomach pain
- Upset stomach
- Vomiting
- Increased hair growth

Felbatol (Felbamate)
- Heartburn
- Vomiting
- Constipation
- Diarrhea
- Weight loss
- Difficulty falling asleep, or staying asleep
- Nervousness
- Drowsiness
- Swelling of the face
- Runny nose
- Differences in menstrual bleeding

Frisium (Clobazam)
- Drowsiness
- Dizziness
- Poor coordination
- Drooling

- Restlessness or aggressiveness
- Anxiety

Gabitril (Tiagabine)
- Confusion
- Difficulty falling asleep or staying asleep
- Difficulty concentrating or paying attention
- Bruising
- Dizziness Itching
- Depression
- Irritability
- Hostility or anger
- Stomach pain
- Increased appetite
- Wobbliness, unsteadiness, or in coordination causing difficulty walking
- Drowsiness
- Lack of energy or weakness
- Nervousness
- Upset stomach
- Speech or language problems
- Painful or frequent urination

Keppra (Levetiracetam)
- Changes in skin color
- Anxiety
- Constipation
- Coordination problems
- Agitation or hostility
- Diarrhea
- Drowsiness
- Nervousness
- Forgetfulness
- Headache
- Dizziness
- Unsteady walking
- Loss of appetite
- Weakness
- Moodiness

- Pain
- Numbness, burning, or tingling in the hands or feet
- Vomiting

Klonopin (Clonazepam)
- Changes in appetite
- Dizziness
- Diarrhea
- Drowsiness
- Blurred vision
- Dry mouth
- Changes in sex drive or ability
- Drowsiness
- Upset stomach
- Constipation
- Difficulty urinating
- Restlessness or excitement
- Frequent urination
- Weakness

Lamictal (Lamotrigine)
- Constipation
- Blurred vision
- Crossed eyes
- Dry mouth
- Rash (most important)
- Difficulty speaking
- Dizziness
- Mood changes
- Difficulty falling asleep or staying asleep
- Difficulty thinking or concentrating
- Cough
- Drowsiness
- Heartburn
- Swelling, itching, or irritation of the vagina
- Diarrhea
- Runny nose
- Irritability
- Loss of balance or coordination

- Missed or painful menstrual periods
- Nervousness
- Problems with ears or teeth
- Double vision
- Stomach, back, or joint pain
- Vomiting

Lyrica (Pregabalin)
- Back pain
- Anxiety
- Confusion
- Difficulty concentrating or paying attention
- Difficulty remembering or forgetfulness
- Bloating
- Dry mouth
- Gas
- Constipation
- Increased appetite
- Headache
- Lack of coordination
- Loss of balance or unsteadiness
- Dizziness
- "High" or elevated mood
- Weight gain
- Muscle twitching
- Nausea
- Speech problems
- Drowsiness
- Weakness
- Uncontrollable shaking or jerking of a part of the body
- Vomiting
- Swelling of the arms, hands, feet, ankles, or lower legs

Mysoline (Primidone)
- Headache
- Changes in appetite
- Uncoordinated
- Drowsiness
- Excitement (in children)

- Irritability
- Upset stomach
- Drowsiness

Neurontin (Gabapentin)
- Anxiety
- Double or blurred vision
- Back or joint pain
- Strange or unusual thoughts
- Fever
- Nausea
- Constipation
- Dry mouth
- Unwanted eye movements
- Diarrhea
- Red, itchy eyes (sometimes with swelling or dis-charge)
- Weight gain
- Drowsiness
- Ear pain
- Vomiting
- Headache
- Heartburn
- Memory problems
- Shaking of a part of your body that you cannot control
- Dizziness
- Drowsiness or weakness
- Unsteadiness
- Swelling of the hands, feet, ankles, or lower legs

Onfi (Clobazam)
- Drowsiness
- Blurred vision
- Dizziness
- Poor coordination
- Drooling
- Restlessness
- Aggressiveness
- Anxiety
- Low blood pressure

- Muscle weakness
- Lack of memory
- Skin rash or itching
- Pounding or irregular heartbeat
- Unusual bleeding or bruising
- Nervousness or irritability
- Unusual fatigue or weakness
- Yellow eyes or skin

Oxtellar XR (Oxcarbazepine extended release)
- Allergic reaction
- Changes in vision
- Confusion
- Fever
- Infection
- Nausea, vomiting
- Trouble with balancing, talking, speaking
- Swelling of the feet or hands
- Trouble passing urine or change in amount of urine
- Unusual bleeding or bruising
- Unusually weak or tired
- Worsening of moods, thoughts, or actions of suicide or dying
- Yellowing of eyes or skin

Peganone (Ethotoin)
- Difficulty breathing
- Wheezing
- Shortness of breath
- Mouth ulcers
- Swollen or painful glands
- Fainting spells or light headed
- Headache
- Poor control of body movements
- Difficulty walking
- Itching
- Loss of seizure control
- Double vision
- Uncontrollable eye movement
- Unusual swelling

- Vomiting
- Fever, sore throat
- Redness, blistering skin
- Yellowing of the eyes or skin
- Skin rash
- Unusual bleeding or bruising
- Pinpoint red spots on skin
- Unusual tiredness or weakness

Phenobarbital (Luminal)
- Agitated
- Clumsiness
- Excessive drowsiness
- Dizziness
- Lightheadedness
- Confusion
- Muscle weakness
- Slowed breathing
- Low blood pressure
- Sleepiness
- Slow heartbeat
- Vomiting
- Headache

Phenytek (Phentoin)
- Constipation
- Headache
- Trouble sleeping
- Swollen lymph nodes
- Nausea
- Vomiting
- Mild nervousness
- Increased heart rate
- Muscle pain
- Unusual Fatigue
- Slurred speech
- Stomach pain
- Numbness or trembling in hands or feet

Potiga (Ezogabine)
- Weak urine stream
- Painful urination
- Confusion
- Aggressive behavior
- Hostile
- Irritable
- Hallucinations
- Paranoia
- Changes in behavior or mood
- Depression
- Panic attacks
- Extreme increase in activity and talking (mania)

Sabril (Vigabatrin)
- Problems walking or feeling uncoordinated
- Dizziness
- Shaking (tremors)
- Joint pain
- Memory problems
- Blurry vision
- Double vision
- Uncontrolled eye movements

Tegretol (Carbamazepine)
- Constipation
- Back pain
- Diarrhea
- Unsteadiness
- Drowsiness
- Dry mouth
- Memory problems
- Headache
- Vomiting
- Dizziness
- Heartburn
- Upset stomach
- Anxiety

Topamax (Topiramate)
- Headache
- Nervousness or irritability
- Shakiness
- Hunger
- Weakness
- Sweating
- Pale skin
- Sudden changes in behavior or mood
- Clumsy
- Jerky movements
- Numbness or tingling around the mouth
- Vertigo
- Lightheaded

Tranxene (Clorazepate Dipotassium)
- Blurred vision
- Difficulty in sleeping or falling asleep
- Depression
- Dizziness
- Drowsiness
- Dry mouth
- Double vision
- Fatigue
- Genital and urinary tract disorders
- Headache
- Irritability
- Lack of muscle coordination
- Mental confusion
- Nervousness
- Tremors
- Skin rashes
- Slurred speech
- Stomach and intestinal disorders
- Tremor

Trileptal (Oxcarbazepine)
- Back pain
- Changes in the way food tastes

- Constipation
- Diarrhea
- Double vision
- Drowsiness
- Dry mouth
- Falling down
- Slowed movements
- Slowed thoughts
- Uncontrollable fast, repetitive eye movements
- Forgetfulness
- Heartburn
- Loss of appetite
- Vision changes
- Stomach pain
- Weight gain
- Swelling, redness, irritation, burning, or itching of the vagina
- Difficulty coordinating movements
- White vaginal discharge
- Difficulty concentrating
- Earache
- Nervousness
- Muscle weakness or sudden tightness
- Uncontrollable shaking of a body part
- Toothache
- Hot flashes
- Mood swings
- Increased sweating
- Speech problems
- Acne
- Nosebleed
- Cold symptoms
- Dizziness

Vimpat (Lacosamide)
- Dizziness
- Nausea
- Vomiting
- Double vision
- Blurred vision

- Fatigue
- Lack of coordination problems
- Vertigo
- General weakness
- Drowsiness
- Memory problems
- Balance problems

Zarontin (Ethosuximide)
- Loss of appetite
- Upset stomach
- Nausea and vomiting
- Heartburn
- Abdominal cramps
- Throat or chest pain
- Weight loss
- Diarrhea
- Drowsiness
- Headaches
- Irritability
- Fatigue

Zebenix (Eslicarbazepine)
- Dizziness
- Drowsy
- Thoughts of harming themselves
- Suicidal thoughts
- Feeling unsteady
- Sensation of spinning or floating
- Nausea
- Vomiting
- Headache
- Diarrhea
- Double or blurred vision
- Difficulty in concentration
- Low in energy, tired
- Shaking
- Clumsiness

Zonegran (Zonisamide)
- Dizziness
- Loss of appetite
- Drowsiness
- Vomiting
- Constipation
- Weight loss
- Confusion
- Upset stomach
- Changes in taste
- Headache
- Irritability
- Dry mouth
- Double vision
- Sneezing
- Difficulty falling asleep or staying asleep
- Burning, pain or tingling in the feet or hands
- Difficulty with memory
- Difficulty focusing eyes
- Runny nose

If you cannot find your medication(s) in this chapter, go to drugs.com

Medications used for status elepticus

- **Ativan** (Lorazepam)
- **Cerebyx** (Fosphenytoin)
- **Diastat** (Diazepam)
- **Dilantin** (Phenytoin)
- **Depakote** (Valproic acid)
- **Depakene** (Valproic acid)
- **Nembutal** (Pentobarbital)
- **Phenytek** (Phenytoin)
- **Valium** (Diazepam)
- **Valrelease** (Diazepam)

"Rescue" medications

The following medications may be used to prevent, stop, or reduce seizure severity.

- **Ativan** (Lorazepam)
- **Diastat** (Diazepam)
- **Klonopin** (Clonazepam)
- **Valium** (Diazepam)
- **Valrelease** (Diazepam)

Status epilepticus and "rescue" medications may have the option of being administered orally, nasally, rectally, and/or IV. Not all seizures or patients respond well or at all to rescue medications.

How to Protect Your Medication Levels

Having a daily medication regimen, which provides consistent seizure control, is not the end of the process in protecting your brain from seizing. Your brain is so sensitive, that a slight change can make the difference between seizures and control.

1. Avoid drinking alcoholic beverages.
2. Do not smoke. It's another good reason to quit!
3. Take your medication as prescribed.
4. Never run out of pills! Request auto refill through your pharmacy; and if necessary, auto delivery. Keep in mind, *every time you get a new written prescription, even if it's just for a refill, you should make sure it remains set up as automatic refill.*
5. If you only have one refill left, contact your doctor for a new prescription immediately. Don't wait! You may not be able to get it filled right away but it'll be ready when you need it.
6. If you miss a dose, do not take it with your next dose! Ask your doctor ahead of time what to do if you miss a pill or dosage of pills.
7. If you've been prescribed a *new medication*, get it filled immediately but wait three days or so before you take it. Keep the extra days worth in another pill container and mark it "extra" or

"back up." Keep track of the earliest refill date possible so you can call it in and keep the extra pills.

8. If possible, take each dose the same time every day.

9. You eat at least three meals a day and probably a snack to regulate hunger pangs, correct? Your brain basically reacts the same way. If your medication is not spread throughout the day as evenly as possible, the balance is thrown off by the dip during mid day which might result in a seizure. The major difference is "snacks" are usually small. But medication is typically more at bedtime in order to get us through the night. If you do not take your medication somewhat equally throughout the day, it's well worth discussing with your doctor.

10. Do not "adjust" your dosage without consulting with your doctor.

11. Use an alarm watch when you're out of your normal routine to prevent forgetting to take it on time or at all.

12. Keep your medication in a dry climate-controlled place. However, for security keep some in your car. Even though it may not be in the ideal climate, it's more important to take the chance that the strength may be compromised rather than have no medication at all.

13. Tell your doctor if you are taking over the counter medication and prescriptions prescribed by another doctor. Other medications can reduce the strength of your AEDs.

14. Make sure the pharmacy has provided your medication as ordered by your doctor (if brand name only).

15. If you use a pill organizer, double check your pills to make sure it's filled correctly before you take them.

16. In case of illness, do not adjust or stop your medication unless otherwise instructed by your doctor.

17. Do not take sinus or cold medications with pseudophedrine. It's a stimulant and works against your antiepileptic medication. Check with your epileptologist or pharmacist to see which expectorant is safest.

18. Do not eat grapefruit or drink the juice! I'm not joking! Grapefruit juice conflicts with the absorption of medication! This includes all medications!

19. Unless the circumstances demand, do not change the brand of medication.

20. Do not take Wellbutrin (anti-depression medication). It may antagonize seizure activity.
21. Avoid using aspartame. Studies suggest aspartame has a connection with seizures in some people with epilepsy.
22. Avoid energy drinks and weight loss supplements.
23. Follow your doctor's advice.
24. Do not take an extra pill when you feel a seizure coming on, it will not help! Some people can use "rescue" medications to prevent an oncoming seizure or even stop a seizure in action. See: *Medications and Possible Side Effects.* Refer to: *Rescue Medications.*
25. *If you find a rescue medication that works, keep some with you at all times.* A small pill holder tucked in your pocket or purse is ideal.
26. Never stop taking your medication without your doctor's assistance.
27. If you have a growth spurt or weight gain, report the information to your doctor.
28. Do not take herbal products without your doctor's knowledge.

The following herbs are known to increase seizure activity:

- Black Cohosh
- Water Hemlock
- Ephedra
- Kava Kava
- Yohimbire
- Guarana
- Mahuang

Nutrition Information

There's no reason that nutritional supplements (multivitamin and calcium) cannot be combined with traditional treatment. They're typically recommended because without question or controversy, those of us who have epilepsy have a definite need to help protect ourselves against medication related damage, and (in theory) against damage caused by the seizures themselves. Therefore, multivitamins and calcium are necessary. However, other supplements may cause adverse reactions if taken improperly or at all. Other than multivitamins and calcium, supplements should be taken with caution and discussed with your doctor.

Look for food sensitivities. Some studies have shown a connection with food allergies and seizures. A health care provider can help you pinpoint possible food allergies. Proof is on record that some food preservatives can trigger seizure activity including MSG. *See the true story at the end of this chapter.*

Be proactive. Take control over your health. It is your doctor's job to inform you but it is your job to take action!

Vitamin B6 is important for normal chemical reactions in your brain. It helps protein to build body tissue and aids in the metabolism of fat. The need for protein intake is relative. As the intake of protein increases, the need for vitamin B6 increases. Deficiency is an associate with seizures in some individuals.

Vitamin B12 is necessary for normal red blood cell formation, tissue, cellular repair, and DNA synthesis. Very low intake can cause nervous system damage. Some AEDs my reduce levels.

Calcium is a major mineral essential for healthy bones and teeth (*must be separate from iron and taken with vitamin D*). Epilepsy increases both men's and women's risk for bone disease therefore calcium is not a luxury, it's a necessity! Adults are generally recommended to take between 1200 – 1800 mg. daily. Discuss the ideal daily dosage *with your doctor.* Take note, you can only absorb 600 mg. at a time.

> ***Certain medications are evidence of reduction in bone health which include but are not exclusive to:***
> - Tegretol, Carbatrol (Carbamazepine),
> - Dilantin (Phenytek)
> - Phenobarbital (Phenytoin)
> - Primidone (Mysoline)
> - Topamax (Topiramate)
> - Depakote (Valproate)

Vitamin D (D3) maintains normal blood levels of calcium and phosphorus. By promoting calcium absorption, it helps to form and maintain strong bones. It also works in concert with a number of other vitamins, minerals, and hormones. Antiepileptic medications can rob your body of its supply of vitamin D! Low levels can set off nervous system disorders.

Vitamin E protects your cells against the effects of free radicals. Antiepileptic medications decrease vitamin E levels. Studies suggest the depletion is significant in its capability to help control seizure activity. A double-blind trial found that adding 400 IU per day, reduced seizure frequency in children without side effects. Other preliminary trials have reported similar results. While some research suggests this effect might exist in adults, a double-blind trial found no effect in adults. It may help reduce the frequency of seizures when used with prescription drugs.

Folic Acid (also known as folate) is important in the production of blood cells. It helps form building blocks of DNA (your body's genetic information), and building blocks of RNA, (needed for protein synthesis in all cells). Rapidly growing tissues, such as those of a fetus, and rapidly regenerating cells, like red blood cells and immune cells, have an excessive need for folic acid. A deficiency results in a form of anemia, which quickly responds to folic acid supplementation.

Women who have the possibility to become pregnant should take folic acid during their childbearing years. Depakote, Dilantin, Tegretol (including XR), Carbatrol, and Phenobarbital can cause a deficiency of folic acid by interfering with the way it is absorbed.

Women who start taking a high dose of folic acid along with Dilantin or Phenytek should have their blood levels checked regularly to see whether the folic acid is causing the medication levels to be lower than expected. Having a low blood level could increase the risk of seizures.

Magnesium is the fourth most abundant element in your brain and is essential in regulating central nervous system excitability. Studies worldwide have shown people who were severely deficient, had increased seizure activity.

Manganese is necessary for a healthy nervous system and optimal immune system. It is responsible for preventing the superoxide free radical from destroying cellular components. In 1963, a link between epilepsy and manganese was found when a study revealed that manganese-deficient rats were more susceptible to seizures than animals with high levels. Other studies have shown that manganese levels are low in blood and hair in epilepsy patients, correlating that those typically having the highest seizure rates showed the lowest levels of manganese.

Melatonin is a hormone produced in the pineal gland located in the center of your brain about the size of a pea! It regulates sleep and may have anti-seizure properties. It is an antioxidant, which means it blocks bad effects from free radicals such as brain damage. There have been a few studies in small numbers of humans which show a significant improvement in seizure control when melatonin is taken in combination with antiepileptic medications.

Omega-3 Fatty Acids play a crucial role in brain function considered essential to human health but your body does not manufacture. Therefore, you must get them through supplements or food.

Research is underway to identify which people with epilepsy are most likely to benefit. Foods high in omega 3 fatty acids include anchovies, mackerel, lake trout, herring, sardines, salmon, black cod, albacore tuna, halibut, wild game, and nuts.

Taurine helps prevent brain cell over-activity. It is utilized in the proper use of potassium and calcium as well as sodium for maintaining cell membrane integrity. It has thought to play a role in the electrical activity of your brain. Several studies have shown positive affects of the anti-convulsive activity of taurine. Another study, which documented epilepsy patients, has shown significantly lower levels of taurine in their blood platelets. There is no agreement on the seizure types or dosage amount for which taurine is most suitable. Deficits of taurine in the brain have been associated with some types of epilepsy.

It may inhibit epileptic seizures in some people. However, the affect appears to be temporary.

Thiamin (previously known as B1) is important for nervous system functioning and has been reported to be associated with seizures in some individuals. It is needed for normal chemical reactions in your brain. Because there is very little Thiamin stored in your body, depletion can occur as quickly as 14 days! Reduced levels in blood and cerebral spinal fluid have been reported in individuals who smoke and have taken Dilantin (Phenytoin) for extended periods. Severe chronic deficiency can result in complications involving your brain.

While reading the supplement deficits and complications, it is obvious medications are a prime factor for most. However, try not to view medication as the "bad guy." After all, most of us have been significantly helped with medication. Yes, they might add complications but they can be corrected. Research every supplement thoroughly then discuss it with your doctor. Together you can overcome the negative aspects of medication. No matter the difficulties caused by medication, learn to appreciate all the qualities they offer.

Herbs

Taking herbs should not be handled lightly with the idea that since they are natural, that makes them safe! For those of us who have epilepsy, that could not only turn out to be far from the truth, it could turn into a disastrous nightmare! It is true that herbs have their healing potential but they may also have ailing potential. The essential oils of many herbal plants contain epileptogenic compounds. So beware of jumping in too fast!

The bottom line is you need to research every herb thoroughly before you make them a part of your daily regimen. However, that is not all! When you feel you are ready, make sure you discuss it with your doctor. Your best chance of bringing the seizures under control and getting on with your life is to follow your doctor's advice. You might think doctors are traditionally medicine-minded only, and that may true for some. However, even those who are against herbal remedies will most likely know which herbs are *confirmed* to be harmful for those of us who have epilepsy.

I do not have a grudge against natural treatments but I would like you to remember, herbs carry some risks including side effects, interactions with medications, and allergic reactions. If claims made about herbal products sound too good to be true, they probably are! When you are ready to start a new approach for better health, enter with caution!

Herbs and Remedies Believed to Aggravate Seizures
(The common name or nickname, is in parentheses)

Artemisia annua (Qing hao, absinthium, sweet wormwood, and annual wormwood)

Bearberry (uva ursi)

Black cohosh (black snakeroot, rattlesnake root, squawroot)

Blue green algae (pond scum, spirulina platensis, spirulina fusiformi)

Borage (bee plant, beebread, borage seed oil, ox's tongue, starflower oil)

Damiana (turnera diffusa, turnera aphrodisiaca)

Ephedra (mahuang, herbal ecstasy)

Evening primrose oil (EPO, night willow herb, fever plant, king's cure-all)

Ginkgo biloba (fossil tree, maidenhair tree, kew tree, yinhsing)

Ginseng (five fingers)

Green tea (Chinese tea, camellia thea)

Guarana (nia sorbilis, guarana, guarana kletterstrauch, guaranastruik, quarane, cupana, Brazilian cocoa, uabano, uaranzeiro)

Horsetail *(equisetum fluviatile,* swamp horsetail) has always been a classic oil to be avoided in epilepsy

Hyssop (hyssopsus)

Lobelia (lobella, asthma weed, eyebright, gagroot, Indian pink, Indian tobacco, pukeweed vomit weed, lobelia berlandieri, and lobelia cardinalis)

Ma huang (ephedra, herbal ecstasy)

Oxygen therapy (oxymedicine, bio-oxidative therapy, oxidative therapy, oxidology, hydrogen peroxide therapy, ozone therapy, ozonolysis, hyper-oxygenation therapies, hyper-oxygenated water, oxymedicine)

Pennroyal (squaw mint, mosquito plant, American pennyroyal, European pennyroyal, mock pennyroyal, squaw balm, tickweed)

Scullcap (huang qin, baikal scullcap, mad-dog herb, helmet flower, hoodwort, Quaker bonnet, ou-gon)

St. John's wort (hypericum perforatum, tipton's weed, klamath weed)

Wormwood (artemisia annua)

As you go on your search for the herb(s) in which you found to be safe and good for your brain, search for sites that have unbiased information. Don't rely on the claims made by someone who is trying to sell a product.

If you believe you found a safe herb, make sure:
- The supply will be readily available.
- It has been *proven* to be safe and effective for people with epilepsy.
- You can rely on the companies or stores consistency, purity, and quality.

- You tell your doctor the name of the herb(s) and daily dose.
- Keep your doctor updated on changes you make concerning your herbal regimen.

If you combine your researched information with your doctor, you'll have the best chance at avoiding unnecessary adverse reactions from herbal therapy. As you go on a search for the right herb(s), remember there is mixed information about some lowering the seizure threshold. As mentioned before, enter with caution!

Dangerous Components

Thujone (Qing hao, absinthium, sweet wormwood, and annual wormwood)

Camphor (cinnamomum camphora, camphor tree or camphor laurel)

MSG food preservative

Neurotox The following products contain neurotox which have convulsant effects which cause neurotoxicity which might in turn cause you to have a seizure:
- Aspartame
- Ammonia
- Carpet cleaning products
- Chlorine
- Combustion products
- Gasoline
- Glues
- Herbicides
- Lacquer
- Municipal sludge
- Paint
- Paint remover
- Paxil
- Pesticides
- Prozac
- Psychiatric medications

- Anti-depressants
- Tranquilizers
- Sleep medications
- Smoke removing agents
- Solvents
- Synthetic carpets
- Welding fumes
- Wood preservatives

In other words, neurotox is everywhere! Since you have epilepsy, neurotox can cause problems. It's obviously not possible to stay away from everything that contains neurotox but it is possible to avoid getting around and using anything you're aware of that contains it.

A Woman's True Story about Her Battle with MSG

I never knew what MSG was before we discovered that it was what caused the seizures. MSG or some form of MSG is in a lot of foods that I used to eat all the time. It is hidden in all kinds of foods and it has many different names, which is what makes it so difficult to avoid. My parents and I asked my neurologists if they had ever heard of MSG or food additives causing seizures. They did not seem to think that was what caused the seizures and just prescribed me to a new medication. Most of the medications would help me for a few months then the seizures would come back, or I would end up allergic to the medication. It was getting incredibly frustrating, and still is.

After I knew the foods I could eat safely, I went a year seizure free. As that year went on, I was crossing off the days, and got more excited every day. I was getting closer to the day that I could finally get my drivers permit. The day that I finally got to one full year felt like the best day of my life. But, within a few days after that one year mark, I did not think of the risk that I was taking when I ate a lot of marshmallows while I was camping. They brought on a grand mal seizure. I was so lucky that I had my sister there with me. She saw me start to fall and guided me to the floor, away from the cast iron stove where I would have hurt myself badly. That seizure was hard for me to deal with.

I had come so far and I made the slightest careless mistake and ruined it for myself. Since then I have had only a few seizures and every time there is never any type of warning sign. Now I found what my triggers are I have learned how to eat right. I really like to look at it as a good thing, because I am avoiding a lot of bad foods that are not really good for anyone. I am so happy that organic and natural foods are becoming very popular because I have a much larger selection now. I would still love to find a medication that could block the seizures, just in case I eat MSG by accident.

I never did grow out of the seizures but I know that one day I will be seizure-free for good. I hope for the chance to be much more independent. I just want to be able to tell people about epilepsy and what mono-sodium glutamate can do. I really hope to help other people that struggle with a similar condition.

Emily Alina

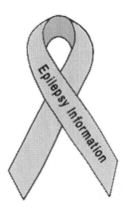

Children's Epilepsy

Epilepsy is one of the most common chronic conditions treated by pediatric neurologists. Twenty percent have an intractable condition. Most children with epilepsy have the same range of abilities and intelligence as other children. However, some children with epilepsy will develop learning difficulties. This may be due to a coexisting condition, such as a brain abnormality, or it might be related to the child's seizure severity. Many times the medication is a contributing factor. When learning difficulties are identified, there are both medical and educational strategies available.

Recognizing Seizures in Children

Not all seizures involve convulsions so it makes them very difficult to recognize, especially in children. Sometimes symptoms are very subtle and often appear to fall within the range of normal childhood behavior. For example, some seizures resemble daydreaming or stumbling and falling. When these seemingly common behaviors occur unusually often or in patterns, they may mean your child's having seizures. Seizures can also be difficult to recognize in young children because they cannot communicate clearly.

"Hidden" signs may include:

- Lack of response for brief periods.
- Sudden episodes of fear with no apparent reason.
- Irritability and unusual sleepiness when wakened.
- Clusters of "jackknife" movements in babies sitting down.
- Dazed behavior.
- Fluttering rapid blinking.
- Frequent complaints about things sounding, looking, smelling, tasting or feeling "funny."
- Repetitive nodding.
- Grabbing movement clusters with both arms in babies lying on their backs.
- Repetitive movements that look unnatural or out of place.
- Short spells of blank staring that look like daydreaming.
- Unusual clumsiness or frequent stumbling.
- Sudden stomach pain followed by confusion and sleepiness.
- Sudden falls for no apparent reason.

The Importance of Early Diagnosis

Recognition of seizures is important for early diagnosis and treatment.

Children whose seizures go unnoticed may face the following problems:

- Behavioral problems. Your child may feel they can't communicate, therefore get frustrated and act accordingly.
- Safety risks. Sudden loss of awareness in certain situations, such as swimming, climbing or riding a bicycle can result in serious injury.
- Learning disabilities. Brief blackouts (loss of consciousness) make it hard to follow the teacher's instructions and keep up with lessons in the classroom.
- Social problems. Your child along with the people they come in contact with don't understand why they're misbehaving or acting unusually out of character. They may be excluded by their peers or personally withdraw socially.

Behavioral Disturbances

Behavioral disturbances can occur in any child whether or not they have epilepsy. Finding the reason for the disturbance in a child with epilepsy can prove to be a difficult task for parents.

The following factors which affect learning in a with epilepsy may also affect their behavior:
- Lack of discipline
- Feeling displaced
- Feeling different (from their peers)
- Low self esteem (from overprotection)

If your child is experiencing behavioral issues you might find it helpful to discuss the issue with their teachers or an epilepsy counselor at the Epilepsy Foundation. They may provide an open door to additional support services. Children with epilepsy should be encouraged to participate in school activities and an after school social life.

Supervisors and teachers are often concerned about caring for a child with epilepsy. Where a risky activity is considered, general restrictions are sometimes wrongly imposed on children with epilepsy. Risks are best assessed on an individual basis. For example, a computer and or video game can trigger seizures in children who experience photosensitive seizures. If your child's trigger is getting overheated, an outdoor warm weather sport will probably not be the correct activity for your child. Instead you can choose an indoor activity with a controlled atmosphere, such as basketball, volleyball, bowling, and many others.

Syndromes

A group of signs and symptoms that, added together, suggest a particular medical condition. In epilepsy, examples of these signs and symptoms would be things like, the age at which the seizures began the type of seizures, whether the child is male or female, and whether they experience difficulties with learning. They can be either symptomatic of underlying brain damage or disease or idiopathic (of unknown cause). In general, idiopathic forms have a better prognosis in terms of both seizure control and eventual remission than do symptomatic forms

Aicardi syndrome is very rare. It does not appear to run in families. It's suspected to be due to spontaneous mutation during conception. It's generally first diagnosed in affected babies between three and five months. There is no cure for nor is there a standard course of treatment. Treatment generally involves medical management of seizures and programs to help parents and children cope with developmental delays. Long-term management by a pediatric neurologist with expertise in the management of infantile spasms is recommended.

Characteristics:
- Abnormally formed bones (backbone and scoliosis).
- Asymmetry of the face (uneven, lopsided).
- Only occurs in girls.
- Caused by brain cysts or other brain abnormalities.
- Physical features are cleft lip and palate.
- Defects of the retina and choroid of one or both eyes.
- Structural abnormalities include partial or completely absent corpus callosum.
- Developmental delay.

Seizure types:
- Infantile spasms (between 3 – 5 months old).
- Generalized tonic-clonic take over when child outgrows infantile spasms.
- Partial motor (less common).
- Complex partial (less common).

Angelman syndrome is a rare condition which used to be called the "happy puppet" syndrome because the children behave as though they are a "puppet-on-a-string." Seizures start between 18 months and two years of age. Eventually seizures will happen in seven or eight out of every ten children with Angelman syndrome.

Characteristics:
- Pointed chin.
- Thin wide mouth.
- Protruding tongue.
- Jerking movements.
- Cheerful mood.
- Bursts of sudden unexplained laughter.
- Fascination for water (usually running water).
- Difficulty understanding language.
- Frequent seizures.
- Seizures may be difficult to treat with AEDs.
- Speech delay.
- Unsteady walking.
- Severe learning difficulties.
- Tongue thrusting.
- Prolonged periods of absence seizures.
- Seizures may initially happen with high temperatures.

Seizure types:
- Absence
- Generalized tonic-clonic
- Myoclonic
- Tonic
- Atonic (less common)

Benign epilepsy of childhood with occipital paroxysms (B.E.C.O.P.)
can start at any age from 15 months to 17 years but usually begins in middle childhood between seven and eleven years of age.

Characteristics:
- Complete or partial visual loss (approximately 50%).
- Sensation of flashing lights (often multicolored spots).
- Visual hallucinations (rare).
- Semi-purposeful movements and behavior (rare).
- Jerking of one side of the body.
- Some children may have seizures as they go from a dark area into a brighter one, or from a well lit area into a dark one.
- Headaches (usually occurring during or after the seizure).

Seizure types:
- Generalized tonic-clonic
- Visual hallucinations
- Photosensitive

Benign myoclonic epilepsy in infancy is a very rare form of epilepsy which in most cases has no identifiable cause and is more common in boys. The seizures begin anywhere from four months to three years of age. Approximately one-third have another family member who either has epilepsy or febrile convulsions. The seizures can start between two and 18 months old but usually start between four and nine months old. The child's development is usually normal and they do not usually have any behavioral problems. This epilepsy syndrome may also run in families.

Characteristics:
- Brief seizures may go unnoticed initially
- head nodding
- loss of balance (rarely fall)
- head drops forward onto their body
- arms tend to move upward and outward
- legs may flex
- eyes roll

Seizure types:
- Complex partial (often occur in clusters from 5 – 10 in each cluster).
- Complex partial may be followed by generalized tonic-clonic.

Benign partial epilepsy in infancy is equally found in boys and girls. Symptoms can start between the ages of two to 18 months but usually start between four and nine months. Out of every 100 children diagnosed with epilepsy before two years of age, five to ten percent will have this syndrome that may run in families.

Characteristics:
- Seizures often occur in clusters of up to 5 – 10 at a time.
- Seizures are typically mild and usually start in the face with the following signs:

- ► Face or cheek twitching.
- ► Tingling, numbness, or unusual sensations in the face or tongue.
- ► Difficulty speaking.
- ► Drooling due to inability to control facial muscles.
- Child stops what they're doing.
- Head may turn to one side.
- May be twitching on one side of the face.
- Learning difficulties.
- Behavioral problems.

Seizure types:
- Complex partial/focal
- Generalized tonic - clonic (typically during sleep)
- Secondarily generalized tonic-clonic
- Absence (blank stares straight ahead or to one side)

Benign Rolandic Epilepsy in Childhood (B.R.E.C.) *a.k.a.* Benign Epilepsy with Centrotemporal Spikes (B.E.C.T.S.) is called 'benign' because it has a good outcome. Nearly all children will outgrow it during puberty. The seizures start in the rolandic area of the brain therefore giving it the name rolandic. It's one of the most common types of epilepsy in children. It affects almost one in five of all children who have epilepsy, both boys and girls. However, boys are a bit more likely to be afflicted. The average onset is six to eight years of age, and often stops around puberty around ages 14 – 18. Children who have close relatives with epilepsy are more commonly affected.

Characteristics:
- Seizures often occur in clusters of up to 5 – 10 at a time.
- Seizures are typically mild and usually start in the face with the following signs:
  - ► Face or cheek twitching
  - ► Tingling, numbness, or unusual sensations in the face or tongue.
  - ► Difficulty speaking
  - ► Drooling due to inability to control facial muscles.

- Child stops what they're doing.
- Head may turn to one side.
- May be twitching on one side of the face.
- Learning difficulties.
- Behavioral problems.

Seizure types:
- Complex partial/focal
- Generalized tonic-clonic (typically during sleep)
- Secondarily generalized tonic-clonic
- Absence (blank stares straight ahead *or* to one side)

Dandy-Walker syndrome is a congenital malformation which occurs in one of every 2,500 live births. It often occurs in infancy, but can also occur in older children. Eighty percent of cases are diagnosed within the first year of life. It typically involves the fourth ventricle of the brain and cerebellum, and the fluid spaces surrounding it. It's regularly associated with disorders of other locations of the central nervous system including absence of the connecting area between the two cerebral hemispheres. Mental and intellectual functions are suppressed in half the patients. The other half may have normal functions.

The degree of symptoms depends on the severity of congenital disease. If severe malformations exist from birth, the signs may worsen at early ages or go unseen until adulthood. Sometimes the only indication can be macrocrania. There is an extreme range of severity.

Characteristics:
- Enlargement of the fourth ventricle
- Partial or complete nonexistence of the cerebellar vermis
- Cyst development in the posterior fossa
- Hydrocephalus
- Macrocrania
- Seizures
- Intracranial pressure in older children, causing vomiting and irritability
- Nystagmus

- Ataxia
- Occiput
- Dysfunction of cranial nerve
- Suppressed motor, speech, and language development (in infancy)
- Delayed development, particularly in motor skills such as crawling, walking, and coordinating movements
- Frequently have muscle stiffness and paralysis of the lower limbs
- Abnormal breathing patterns
- Possible structural abnormalities:
  - ► kidney and urinary abnormalities
  - ► Malformations of the heart, face, limbs, fingers, and toes
  - ► Cleft lip and palate
  - ► Extra fingers or toe
  - ► Fused fingers or toes

Seizure type:
- Generalized tonic-clonic

Doose Syndrome *a.k.a.* Juvenile Myoclonic Astatic Epilepsy of Early Childhood (M.A.E.) is an extremely rare genetic disorder affecting one to two percent of children with epilepsy. It commonly starts around 18 months to two years old. It usually affects children that have previously developed normally, afflicting more boys than girls. In approximately one third of the cases, another family member (immediate or extended) may have seizures but not always the same kind. It's typically resistant to medication which makes it hard to treat. However, as researchers learn more about M.A.E., new options become available, and the outcome is more favorable.

Characteristics:
- Astatic
- Cognitive problems
- Dyspraxia
- Disarthria
- Slow speech
- Seizure severity ranges from mild to severe

Seizure types:
- Myoclonic and/or myoclonic-astic
- Febrile convulsions
- Generalized tonic-clonic
- Atonic
- Absence
- Non-convulsive status elepticus

Dravet syndrome *a.k.a.* Severe Myoclonic Epilepsy of Infancy (S.M.E.I.) is a severe form of epilepsy. Thirty to eighty percent of cases, caused by defects in a gene required for the proper function of brain cells. The symptoms begin during the first year of life.

Development is normal prior to the onset of seizures. Affected infants develop either generalized or unilateral clonic seizures. Myoclonic jerks and partial seizures usually appear later. Psychomotor retardation and other neurologic deficits occur in affected children.

The first seizure type that appears is a clonic seizure, either generalized or unilateral, often changing sides. These seizures may be either brief or long in duration. In many cases, the first seizure appears in association with a fever. The febrile seizures in these cases often recur in six to eight weeks, and may be prolonged, leading to status epilepticus.

Later in the course, the seizures may recur without rise of body temperature. These convulsive seizures, carefully analyzed with video e.e.g. recordings performed along the course, are polymorph. They can be clearly generalized, clonic, and tonic-clonic, or unilateral, and hemiclonic.

Characteristics:
- Poor development of language and motor skills.
- Hyperactivity.
- Difficulty relating to others.
- Appears during the first year of life with frequent febrile seizures.
- Other types of seizures typically arise later, including myoclonic and complex partial.
- Status elepticus.

Seizure types:
- Febrile convulsions (15 – 30 minutes, or longer)
- Tonic-clonic
- Myoclonic astatic
- Photosensitive
- Generalized clonic
- Generalized tonic-clonic
- Partial
- Hemiclonic
- Unilateral
- Status elepticus

Janz syndrome *a.k.a.* Juvenile Myoclonic Epilepsy (JME), Adolescence Myoclonic Epilepsy is a common type of epilepsy. Doctors are becoming more aware of this syndrome. It's estimated that about 10% of cases of epilepsy, and perhaps more are juvenile myoclonic epilepsy. Because children and their parents may not realize that myoclonic jerks in the morning are abnormal and may not tell their doctor about them, it's not certain how many children have juvenile myoclonic epilepsy. In some cases the child had febrile seizures or childhood absence seizures. It's more likely in children who have family members with generalized epilepsy. It usually begins between eight to 18 years old or sometimes in early adulthood in people with a normal range of intelligence. It afflicts girls more than boys. In girls, it may be associated with menstruation. In most cases it can be well controlled with medication but must be continued throughout life.

Characteristics:
- Jerks with sudden brief muscle contractions on one or both sides of the body.
- Jerks mainly involve neck, shoulders, and upper arms.
- If the child is holding an object, it can be thrown across the room.
- Occasionally the jerks may affect the legs or even the entire body which may cause the child to fall down.
- Child remains conscious.
- Jerks usually occur after awakening in the morning or after a nap.
- Jerks can interfere with normal activities like brushing teeth and eating breakfast.

- The child and parents may believe jerks are normal, or that they are due to clumsiness or nervousness.
- The myoclonic jerks can be triggered by:
  - ► Awakening (nearly 15 – 60 minutes after)
  - ► Television
  - ► Video games
  - ► Lack of sleep
  - ► Tired
  - ► Stress
  - ► Excitement
  - ► Fasting
  - ► Drugs
  - ► Alcohol
  - ► Menstruation
  - ► Flashing or flickering lights (about 1/3 patients)
  - ► Decision making (concentrating)
  - ► In 76% of children, seizures are triggered by:
- drawing
- writing
- calculating
- In some cases, the seizures do not cause visible movements. They are a shock-like sensation inside their body.
- Once the child starts experiencing jerks from myoclonic jerks for several years, they usually start to have generalized tonic-clonic seizures.
- The child may be able to tell from the myoclonic jerks that a tonic-clonic seizure is about to happen.
- Intelligence remains normal.
- Some children may have poor social adjustment.

Seizure types:
- Myoclonic (defining symptom)
- Tonic-clonic
- Absence
- Generalized tonic-clonic

Landau–Kleffner syndrome *a.k.a.* Infantile Acquired Aphasia, Acquired Epileptic Aphasia, or Aphasia with Convulsive Disorder is a rare disorder occurring in normal children affecting twice as many boys than girls. It develops in children typically between the ages of three to seven years who lose previously achieved speech and language skills. Some children recover while others have significant language impairments that persist.

Characteristics:
- Behavioral changes.
- Seizures regress over time.
- Highly abnormal e.e.g.
- The child who develops the inability to speak also shows trouble understanding what is said to them.
- On rare occasions, a severe behavioral disorder with autistic and psychotic characteristics may develop.

Seizure types:
- Tonic-clonic
- Complex partial

Lennox Gastaut syndrome (L.G.S.) is a rare syndrome which begins between two to six years old yet doesn't exclude the the possibility that seizures can start before two years old and after six. It may be very strong and become more difficult to control over time. It's often accompanied by developmental delay, and psychological and behavioral problems. Due to type and frequency of seizures, sudden falls and injuries are likely. The child usually wears a helmet.

Characteristics, seizure types:
- Broad range of seizures (larger than any other syndrome).
- Daily multiple seizures are typical.
- Frequently have slowed or arrested psychomotor development and behavior problems.

Seizure types:
- Atonic
- Tonic, most frequent type (90% are nocturnal)

- Absence
- Tonic-clonic
- Myoclonic
- Complex partial
- Status elepticus (usually nonconvulsive)

Ohtahara syndrome is very rare and starts before three months of age as early as the first ten days of life. Most babies have an underlying structural brain abnormality which may be genetic in origin or due to brain damage before or around the time of birth.

Characteristics:
- Developmental impairments
- Myoclonus
- Mental retardation
- Reduced muscle tone
- Psychomotor retardation

Seizure types:
- Tonic spasms
- Partial motor
- Generalized tonic-clonic
- Infantile spasms

Rasmussen syndrome *a.k.a.* **Rasmussen Encephalitis** is a rare form of brain malfunction which most commonly affects children ages three to eleven years old. The cause is unknown. The brain cells in one hemisphere become inflamed and swollen. There's no evidence of infection in most cases however, an occasional virus is detected. It's possible for a virus to trigger an antibody response in the brain causing inflammation. Malfunctioning of the brain is caused by the inflammation which in turn causes frequent seizure activity. The seizures are usually very difficult to control with medication.

Characteristics:
- Seizures are often the first symptom to appear.
- Develop weakness on one side of the body 1 – 2 years after the seizures start.
- As seizures pursue, weakness worsens.

- Can lead to permanent damage of the nerve cells.
- Intellectual dysfunction.

Seizure type:
- Simple partial motor

Rett syndrome is due to a genetic abnormality found in the X chromosome. Rett syndrome affects approximately every 10,000 – 12,000 girls. Boys are rarely affected but are always more severe than girls. The seizures nearly always start within the first months of life and are often extremely difficult to treat. Girls may show normal development until between six and 30 months of age. Girls have periods of slow or rapid breathing which are sometimes associated with fainting and mistaken for epileptic seizures.

Characteristics:
- Development slows down and may reverse
- Become less interested in play
- Lose the ability to speak
- Become irritable and scream for no obvious reason
- Stop using hands purposefully
- Move hands repetitively

Seizure types:
- Generalized tonic-clonic
- Tonic
- Absence
- Infantile spasms
- Myoclonic

Sturge-Weber syndrome is a rare condition indicated at birth by seizures and accompanied by a large birthmark on the forehead and upper eyelid. The birthmark varies in color from light pink to deep purple caused by abnormal blood vessels on the surface of the brain. The seizures that begin in infancy may worsen with age. Convulsions usually happen on the side of the body opposite the birthmark and vary in severity. There may also be muscle weakness on the same side.

Some children will have developmental delays and mental retardation. Most will have glaucoma (increased pressure within the eye) at birth or develop it later. The increased pressure within the eye can cause the eyeball to enlarge and bulge out of its socket. It rarely affects other body organs, and is not associated with heredity. It's very uncommon to have more than one child with Sturge-Weber syndrome in the same family. The seizures start anywhere from birth to one year old. Learning difficulties occur in two out of three children. The more frequent and severe the seizures are the greater severity of the learning difficulties.

Characteristics:
- "Port wine" birthmark
- Resistant to anti epileptic drug (AED) treatment
- Weakness on one side of body
- Weakness may worsen with growth

Seizure types:
- Generalized tonic-clonic
- Atonic (drop attacks)
- Myoclonic
- Infantile spasms
- Status elepticus

West's syndrome (infantile spasms) is a specific type of seizure seen in an epilepsy syndrome of infancy and early childhood. The onset is predominantly in the first year of life typically between three to six months. Infants may have dozens of clusters ranging from two to one hundred spasms at a time. They may also have dozens of clusters and several hundred spasms per day. The seizures usually stop by age five but are often replaced by other seizures.

Characteristics:
- Suddenly bend forward
- Stiffening of arms, legs, and body
- Arching torso (sometimes)
- Usually begin seconds after arousal from sleep

Seizure type:
- Infantile spasms

My Little One

For my little one,
I cry, I beg, I plead, I pray
That one day the seizures will go away.
Just when you think the storm has passed,
It sneaks back up on you oh so fast,
With no warning at all
As I watch my little one fall
The feeling of despair
Thinking this is just not fair!
As you awake from your sleep
My emotions so deep
These seizures I know we will beat.
I ask why you?
Why my child with that beautiful smile?
I try to understand why God's plan
Was to put this special child in my hands
I guess He knew I'd be your biggest fan!
I will never lose sight of hope
As each day I learn how to cope,
Never knowing when the next storm will hit
Next to you, is where I will always sit.
My promise to my little one is this,
No matter how hard the road we travel or how scary it may seem,
We will always be on the same team!
I will stand by you forever
I give up on you, never!
My unconditional love for you
Will always remain true!

*Thank you, Wanda Musto for sharing this beautiful poem
and a window into your heart.*

True Stories about Our Little Ones

Jayden, a precious baby boy was born into the world with excitement and anticipation for a bright and happy future. Brandy had just come home from work after her second week back from maternity leave. Her husband's aunt, who was babysitting two and a half month old Jayden, reported he had been a little "fussy." Brandy was getting concerned because he kept "whining." He started opening and closing his mouth in an odd way over and over. So in an attempt to keep him from doing that, she put her finger on his chin.

She said, "My first reaction was to make him stop. I was a little panicky. I always second guess myself, so I thought, 'Did I see what I really think I saw?'" Her second reaction was to yell for her husband who was outside. She stated, "He knew by my voice, something was wrong. And I shouted, 'I think Jayden's having a seizure!' Everything happened so fast. I called 9-1-1 and they asked, 'How do you know it was a seizure'? I responded, 'Because it wouldn't stop! I have three other children, and I've never experienced something like this!"

The ambulance came and the paramedics asked Brandy questions like, "Has he been sick? Did he have a fever?" Then they took Jayden to the hospital in the ambulance. But since he wasn't seizing at the time of arrival, they put Brandy and Jayden in the waiting room. After a long wait, they took him to get a CT scan. Approximately five hours later, the doctor told Brandy the test result was "normal." She said, "Tell me what happened because babies don't seize like that! So, I don't know what you think you saw. You can go home now, and if it happens again come back." Just as she said that, Jayden's left arm went up and started shaking. Brandy wasn't sure about the first one but she knew that one was a seizure for sure.

The nightmare continued as Jayden continued to have seizures. Directly after Jayden's six week stay in the hospital when he was just six months old, Brandy recognized the necessity of documenting Jayden's seizure activity so she designed a chart.

The doctors tried to control the seizures using a wide range of medications. Over time, he was put through a battery of tests which included MRI, CT scan, PET scan, etc. Jayden was experiencing really long convulsions. He was diagnosed as having a metabolic disorder of unknown cause. However, unless he had electrodes implanted on both sides of his brain, he would not be considered a candidate for surgery. Brandy didn't want to put him through that extreme yet because the doctors could not guarantee he would be able to go forward with surgery.

But Jayden did have a video e.e.g. The "head honchos" were focusing on the left side of his brain for resection surgery. Brandy said she would consider that even though it could cause him loss of peripheral vision and partial paralysis on one side. She would consider that an option because she reasoned the side effects from the surgery are nothing compared to seizure control. If he had seizure control he would be able to learn and make progress.

Brandy made it clear how she viewed doctors when she stated, "Women doctors are much better because they aren't afraid to say, 'I don't know but I will find out!" She was simply disgusted with the care he was receiving. He was seen by many doctors and some believed it was a lost cause trying to help him and one told her to quit! Determined and highly emotional Brandy, made it clear, "I have a special needs child. I push and push and push until I get what I want!" She made it clear, "I will never give up on him!"

She talked to many people on her "journey." Along the way, she met numerous people. She met moms that she wanted to shake and ask them, "What are you doing?" She was amazed regarding the available information she got by talking to social workers, moms, teachers, therapists, etc.

Jayden tried everything, all the medications and everything imaginable. He's gone through the "lists." It came to a point when the doctors knew they had to do something or all the medications were going to kill him. There were only two options left. One was a medication that had not been FDA approved.

The doctors were resistant about Jayden trying it because they knew it could cause irreversible damage, and is the reason it was taken off the market since. So that left them with one option, the vagus nerve stimulator. However, one of his doctor's was not a fan of the VNS. He thought Jayden was too small and it simply wouldn't work on him. He wanted to try other options. However a decision for a VNS was won over. So Jayden had a VNS implanted in August 2006. The implantation was somewhat "easy." Jayden only needed Tylenol to manage his pain.

Just one day after it was implanted, it was turned on! Brandy said, "The original plan was to wait a week. Typically they wait a week until it heals but they decided to turn it on to see what would happen. In Jayden's case it was instantaneous! He was alert in a couple days! They'd turn it up a little at a time until they got it where they wanted. Then they sent him home! Brandy said with excitement, "The VNS gave him a better quality of life. I couldn't be happier with where we are with him."

Jayden's improvements due to the VNS:

- He doesn't have postictal difficulties. Before the VNS he'd have a "big" seizure with rectal Diastat. But after the VNS, he has faster recovery.
- He doesn't show a tired feeling. Now when he has a seizure, they can "go on their way."
- He's more alert.
- The seizures are controlled better instantly. In the "beginning" a short seizure was 20 minutes to a half hour. To stop them he would be pumped with medication, and taken in the ambulance with an IV, pumped with more medication and sent home for Brandy to take care of him.
- The seizures are shorter!
- Brandy was thrilled to mention that an ambulance has not been needed since!

Six months after the VNS was implanted Jayden started losing the small amount of skills like sitting up with minimal support and head control. Brandy kept seeing him make a "weird" face followed by a smile. Sometimes he would throw his arms up in the air. She complained to the doctors over a three month period but to no avail. So she took him to the doctor so they could see Jayden's "activity" first hand.

Initially they believed it was due to the fact he was growing so fast and having a hard time keeping up. But Brandy didn't have trouble keeping up with documenting the "events" as she started to count how many episodes he was having. She went to his doctor and reported he had 30 in one day and demanded an e.e.g.!

After the e.e.g., Brandy woke up to her next nightmare because she received the news that Jayden was experiencing infantile spasms. She was devastated. She felt the VNS was the promise of a flourishing future, and she was sure they were on the right road. She was getting tired of the negative always creeping back in. But Brandy won't let negativity steal her joy. She is a strong woman who doesn't just see the epilepsy in her little boy's life. She recognizes the full picture. She said with compassion, "God gave me this child for a reason. I'll take the good with the bad. He's a blessing in my eyes. So in the end, epilepsy is an actual symptom of what is wrong with Jayden, with a diagnosis still unclear. But we will keep moving forward."

They tested for many things. He went to two different medical centers. But Brandy's not exhausted, she said, "I'm all ears when the medical team is doing their work." People started preparing Brandy, that when Jayden turned three, he needed to move on and go to school. Brandy had been dreading his first day however it wasn't so bad after all! His daddy took an early lunch and met them at the school. A friend who also has a special needs child joined them, and they comforted each other.

So Jayden started special needs preschool when he was three years old! The family started a new adventure which has proven to be exciting especially looking forward to how well Jayden will be doing after six months of schooling!
Brandy, Stockton CA

So far Cody leads a pretty normal life. He was born with epilepsy. The seizures came from the left temporal and frontal lobes. He had petite and complex partial seizures. He was having so many petite seizures a day that it was interfering with learning speech. When he was 18 months old, he was diagnosed with a brain tumor on the right side of his brain (thalamus and basal ganglia). Then he had his first grand mal that went into status epilepticus. His medications were switched which has done wonders for him. The only time he has a seizure now is when they try to wean him off the medicine or when he outgrows his dosage.

After his last e.e.g. they decided he will probably never be off medicine. He still has seizure activity from the left temporal and frontal lobes. But they are also coming from the right temporal lobe where his incision was to remove the tumor. He has never had a normal e.e.g. He has been seizure-free for four months now. The time length before that was three years! He doesn't let this stand in his way from doing the things any seven year old child would do. He plays sports and rides bikes, etc. Despite everything, he is the happiest kid I have ever known! You can visit Cody on the web at codybugs-talltales.com. *Jenn*

Dallas was hospitalized for a video e.e.g. for over 48 hours. We got a lot of information without having to take him off any medication. To all who told me, it wasn't going to be easy keeping a kid down in bed for any length of time, YOU WERE RIGHT! I think that was the worst part of it all! The first day with him on the e.e.g. didn't really show anything. But about 1 ½ hours after going to sleep, boy did this kid's brain start acting up!

He has left temporal and frontal lobe seizures. He has spike wave events and seizures and they are very active. They don't make him have any external shaking or twitching, which really surprised the doctor and neuroscience department. They kept calling me to ask why I wasn't pushing the seizure button! I told them he wasn't doing anything on this end!

The doctor increased his medication big time! Dallas had an MRI and spinal tap. The fluid was sent to four different places to see if we

can get more answers, like why he's having these type of seizures, and what more we can do for him. The possible treatment is different mixtures of medication. If nothing works, then we'll talk surgery. That's if all else fails! This doctor finally realizes what I have been telling him. So now we might finally get somewhere.
K. Stokes, Sacramento CA

When I gave birth to my beautiful little girl Taylor, everything was just perfect. However, Taylor had her first grand mal seizure approximately one month after her first birthday party. My life along with hers changed forever. Prior to this day, I never really knew what a seizure was nor had I ever seen one. It was terrifying. I did not know what was happening to my baby. I called 9-1-1 and an ambulance arrived. It was then that I learned that my baby was having a seizure. I was beside myself in disbelief.

One month later, my daughter was diagnosed with epilepsy. Everything just worsened from that day on. Taylor had seizure after seizure. I took her to see many different doctors, and she tried several different medications. We had no success with controlling the seizures. At around six years old, she had a vagus nerve stimulator (VNS) implanted with the attempt to control the seizures. We had no success. By the time she was eight years old, she was at her worst, having back-to-back seizures.

Taylor was slipping away fast. Every effort seemed hopeless. The doctor we were seeing at that time felt Taylor was in a critical life-threatening state, so he recommended that I seek a second opinion. I took Taylor to my hometown of New York City to find a doctor.

We later scheduled an appointment at a Comprehensive Epilepsy Center. We met with a wonderful neurologist. Following our first visit with him, we were scheduled to have Taylor admitted into the hospital for video e.e.g. monitoring for one week. After the testing was over, Taylor was finally properly diagnosed with doose syndrome.

With the correct diagnosis after seven years and a change in her medications, I am thrilled to say Taylor is now one year seizure-free! I cannot express enough gratitude towards her doctor for giving Taylor her life back, and also giving me my little girl back!

Taylor is a beautiful nine year old child with such a big heart. She was so brave through it all. Although she has cognitive delays, she is a typical nine year old little girl who loves to go to school, watch cartoons, play with her little brother, swim, read, etc.

The best advice I can give to other parents who have children with epilepsy is to never give up hope. My love for my child gave me the strength and persistence to never give up. Today I live day to day and know that this is a disability Taylor will carry throughout her life. But for now, we have won the battle. I have learned so much throughout this ordeal. I have learned how fragile life is and how important my faith is. I have learned to be more compassionate towards others and enjoy every single day with my family. God bless all the families who have children with epilepsy.
W. Musto, Myrtle Beach SC

Jimmie is our only child. We married late in life. We waited a full year before trying to have a baby to no avail. The problem was me. I took fertility drugs for six months with no results. Then I took a dye test. One ovary was completely blocked. So the doctor referred us to a fertility specialist, who promised he could get us pregnant within three months! We were pregnant with our little miracle! It was a normal pregnancy. I loved being pregnant. But I am older, and I have high blood pressure. Of course my blood pressure was better pregnant than it was before I was pregnant but I was still considered high risk.

At the end of my pregnancy, I was having non-stress tests weekly. Jimmie was due on July 3. On June 20, I had the non-stress test and the technician noted that the amniotic fluid had dropped from 9.8 to 9.3, whatever that means! She requested I talk to the doctor about increasing the non-stress testing to twice a week. I had an ultrasound a couple days later. They wanted to know Jimmie's size to determine if he should be delivered because I was quite large. He was actually small, but the amniotic fluid was down to 3.8. They sent me directly to labor and delivery to be induced.

He was born the next day via emergency c-section because he was quite stubborn! He would not turn face down or go any lower in the birth canal. His heart rate was dropping during pushing. His apgar was great @ 9.9. He became slightly jaundiced but that corrected itself without medication.

He was small but not too small at 6 lb ½ oz. He was simply the most beautiful baby I had ever seen! He developed normally for the first 4 ½ months of his life. Then I began to notice very brief repetitive episodes at feeding and bath times. He would look up to the right with a slight jerking motion in his torso. To me the episodes looked like his brain switching off and back on. He did not appear to notice them at all. When they occurred while he was playing, he simply resumed playing as if nothing had happened!

I told my husband about the episodes. He thought I was talking about Jimmie just looking at something else and dismissed it. But I was not so convinced. When he was home one evening, I made him come and watch Jimmie in the bath. When one of the episodes occurred, I pointed at Jimmie and said, "There! See that?" He stood there for a second and then said very quietly, "Well that is something!"

So we got our video camera out and video-taped him as we fed him and changed his clothes to get him ready for bed. We caught a few episodes. The next day I called the pediatrician and got an appointment for the following day. We both went and showed the video. The doctor was also convinced we were seeing seizures. He referred us to a Children's Hospital in Chicago to see a pediatric neurologist.

Jimmie had an e.e.g. The results were devastating. His pattern was called hypsarrhythmia. It, along with the seizures, gave us the diagnosis of infantile spasms which, while it sounds benign, is actually a very devastating diagnosis. Most children are severely delayed. Most children will develop some other form of devastating epilepsy once the infantile spasms spontaneously disappear.

Most commonly the epilepsy progresses to Lennox Gastaut Syndrome. The prognosis is not good. It is better for kid's whose infantile spasms are cryptogenic or idiopathic in origin. So far, Jimmie's infantile spasms are idiopathic. But we are still testing for possible causes.

Despite the improved chances for a good prognosis, the seizures are not affected by drug therapy. His diagnosis has been upgraded to mixed seizure disorder with intractable seizures and status post infantile spasms.
L. Mathes, Sterling IL

Kaitlin was diagnosed with Refractory Complex Partial Epilepsy at age seven. Her epilepsy eventually progressed, and she was diagnosed with *Juvenile Myoclonic Epilepsy* when she was thirteen. She is currently fifteen and suffers from migraines, grand mals (generalized tonic-clonic,) myoclonic, and petit mal seizures. She has no warnings in the form of auras. After a seizure, she is very irritable, tired, and lethargic. She experiences myoclonic seizures nightly. She never gets a break from them. She never has a chance to relax and breathe. She wakes up tired every morning.

Seizures are just a part of Kaitlin's battle. She had problems with her kidney functions due to her medications which included a kidney stone at the age of fourteen. With her additional side effects, her doctor's have been closely watching her liver function which involves monthly blood work. She has so much stress in her life, that it causes trauma, anxiety, memory loss, increased sensitivity, and fear of being alone.

She's taking two antiepileptic medications. One causes moodiness so she has to take another medication to offset the effect. Even with the medication she has very erratic mood swings which she does not have any control over. Because of her unrelenting side effects, she has a special educational plan at school.

She has to wear blue tinted glasses to protect her eyes from the florescent lights, in addition to help her process the information she is reading effectively. Our physician recommended the colored glasses once we found out that color effectively helped Kaitlin. Our physician recommends this to people to try color variations from red, salmon, yellow, and green. Blue worked successfully for Kaitlin!

Kaitlin doesn't have the luxury to enjoy typical teenager activities such as going to "sleep over's" at her friends. She doesn't even "sleep over" at a family member's home. She struggles educationally. She does not like to ask for the help she has been offered because she doesn't want to appear different. She does not use the tools set up for her in the 504 plan. She cooks and goes on roller coasters rides! She loves golden retrievers and sloths.

She has lost friends after they witnessed a seizure. They will not even speak to her now, for fear of not knowing what epilepsy and seizures are. Regardless of her epilepsy, she enjoys swimming and skateboarding. She is a risk taker. She likes to read and write poetry, and listen to music. She likes to star gaze for hours! In other words, she's a normal teenager who just happens to have epilepsy. *Alison Y, Palm Bay FL*

John and I have been blessed with three children, Gianna, Ethan and Maya. Our Son, Ethan was born on March 8, 2003. God had a plan in store for him the day he was born. He was a healthy baby boy with no signs of medical problems. We were so happy when we saw our little boy. When the doctor handed me my son I thought he was so precious. I loved my bundle of joy so much! John was visualizing them already throwing a football back and forth! He was looking forward to the future, not knowing what was in store.

Growing up, Ethan developed normally. We did everything that a mother and father should do for their child. Everything seemed to be going perfect. To hear his first word and to see him take his first step were the best feelings that any parent can experience. As time went along, Ethan was a typical one-year-old, making a mess with his toys and enjoying playing with his sister, Gianna.

Before I knew it, he was already turning two. He loved to watch Elmo on TV. He would laugh so much every time he heard Elmo's voice! By this time Ethan was curious about his surroundings, he would get into Grandma Rosie's cookbooks and tear them! Even though they were part of her collection, she never had the heart to get mad at him!

As time went along, he was already turning three. Boy was he a handful! He was in his spider-man phase! Anything and everything had to be spider-man! He did the moves and sounds of the web shooting out! It was funny to see him pretend that he was the "real" spider-man. From this time on life would not be the same and we did not know if it ever would.

Miracles are when God reveals himself when you believe in Him. You gain an awareness of Him. You see everything in a new light. He shows us His great power through the trials and tribulations of life. April 6, 2006, is the day that we will never forget. It was around 8:30 a. m. and we were getting ready for the day. Ethan was standing behind Yvette (his mommy) as she was getting Maya dressed. He was so quiet that she turned around, at that moment she saw him on the floor shaking. He was not breathing and his eyes were rolled back.

All of a sudden, he was turning blue. She thought he was suffocating. I can remember it so clearly. All I could hear is Yvette screaming, "John, Ethan is not moving he won't get up." I got there to see him very unresponsive in Yvette's arms. As I panicked, I took Ethan from her not knowing what was happening. I tried everything that I could to wake him up or get him to breathe.

I was so scared that I did not know what was happening to our son. (*When I am afraid, I will trust in GOD; Psalms 56:3*) By then, the ambulance and medical technicians had arrived. They told us that Ethan was having a seizure, and there was nothing we could do but let the seizure pass. That was the hardest thing to see Ethan go through.

We took Ethan to the doctor, so he could evaluate and make sure that he was fine. But since Ethan never experienced this before, his doctor drew concern. He sent us to a Children's Hospital to meet with a pediatric neurologist who preformed an e.e.g. and prescribed seizure medication temporarily so that he would not have another seizure. However, that was not the case. Weeks after the first seizure, Ethan had reoccurring seizures episodes ranging from drop seizures, petit mal seizures, and grand mal seizures. So from there on, I knew what to expect each time he would have a seizure. It was scary but I knew he would be okay.

We began seeing two neurologists on a daily basis in hope that they could find a cure for him. Each time something went wrong with Ethan, he did not look well. The doctor was always there for us with an open door. He took care of Ethan as best as he could medically. Every time we went to see the other neurologist, he would always tell us that Ethan was giving him gray hair because he could not find a cause for the seizure activity! Therefore he scheduled a MRI (in 2006.) He wanted to see if he could find any answers. And he did find something!

He told us that Ethan has abnormal white matter in his brain. He said he had other doctors from other prestigious hospitals evaluate the MRI images. They told us the extent of the abnormal white matter showed that Ethan should not be developing or functioning as a normal child should.

How do we as parents cope with something so tragic? We could not understand why this was happening to him. (*Trust in the Lord with all your heart and lean not on your own understanding; in all your ways acknowledge Him, and He will make your paths straight.* Proverbs 3:5-6)

Over time, his body became frail due to the amount of seizure activity that occurred repeatedly. He was hospitalized three times in hopes that the doctor could make him well. Ethan went through numerous testing, and the conclusions that were found were that he had a probable seizure disorder but the cause was still unknown.

In April 2007, I met with the neurologist and he mentioned that he had a resource that he wanted Ethan to see. But the doctor he wanted Ethan to see would be far away, and asked if we would be willing to travel out of town in order to seek medical attention. He gave me his number to schedule an appointment. I did but the next available appointment wasn't until September 12, 2007.

So as time passed, Ethan's condition was worsening. He was having frequent seizures, and had to wear a helmet at times to protect him from injury. It hurt me to see him that way. (*I can do all things through Christ who strengthens me. Phil 4:13*) Often at times I would just cry, and ask GOD why was this happening to him. He was just a little boy and did not deserve to go through this at such a young age.

In May 25, 2007 was the day Ethan took a turn for the worst. He was taking a nap, and we didn't hear him get up. My dad, John, and I heard a loud thump in the restroom. We ran to see what happened. Ethan was using the restroom when he had a seizure. He fell and hit his mouth and teeth on the toilet. John and I grabbed him and took him to the Medical Center. We didn't know the extent of the damage, until the doctors cleaned him up. Two teeth were pushed into the gum and he busted his lip. We brought him home, and he wasn't the same. He didn't want to walk and he lost his appetite.

May 28, 2007, I took him to his neurologist. He immediately got on the phone with another doctor. They were talking for a while. Then the doctor came into the room with tears in his eyes. He told me that the doctor was arranging for us to go to distant city as soon as possible. From that moment on, I was so scared. I was told to take him to Children's Hospital, and from there they were going to transport us to another Children's Hospital. As soon as we arrived to the medical center, the medical team began preparing us for our journey. It was just a matter of time.

It was about 6 p. m. On May 29, and the medical team came into the room, to tell us that Ethan was ready to go. We were told at first that we would be transported by helicopter or ambulance and only one parent could go along. So I told John that I wanted to go with him. However, as we were making our way down, the medical team said that we would be going by jet. Someone anonymously donated the use of the jet that would be transporting us!

I turned to the Lord in this time of need when my son was at his worse. I placed my son under His care and humbly asked that he restore him to good health as we began our journey. Upon arriving at the children's hospital, he was immediately placed in the epilepsy care unit and put on seizure monitors. From there, we met with numerous pediatric neurologists and were asked many questions about Ethan's medical condition.

The following day we met with the epilepsy specialist. He evaluated Ethan and went over numerous notes from his doctor back home, and reviewed the tests that were done. He mentioned that he was not concerned about the abnormal white matter because he probably was born with it. He told us that it caused no problem and was not linked to the seizure activity. He took him off one of his medications and put him a new one. We were told that Ethan should get better but it was all up to GOD.

We came back home and he was getting a little better. We prayed each and every day that the Lord would make him well. We had numerous supports through family, friends, church organizations, and people we had never met that lifted Ethan in prayer. *Whatever you ask in prayer with faith you will receive.* Matthew 21:22

June 4, 2007, was the last time that Ethan had a seizure and it has been 8 ½ months to the day of being seizure-free! I thank GOD for making Ethan well and giving him a second chance at life. GOD truly has a purpose for Ethan, and we are blessed and thankful for the miracle that He has preformed right before our eyes. We met with the doctors, and they all stated that medically there is no explanation for Ethan's rapid recovery! That he is truly a miracle of GOD!!! *With God all things are possible.* Matthew 19:26
Y. Navarro, Poteet TX

Bailey was at a point where he was suffering from Todd Paralysis on a daily basis. He would become completely paralyzed in his right leg, and almost totally in his right arm. I thought he may have been having strokes or something. It was very severe. He was missing weeks of school.

There was no warning. He would wake from a seizure and try to get up to use the bathroom, and fall flat on his face. It was lasting for up to four hours a day, sometimes less. It was not only scary but very upsetting to him and very confusing, never knowing if it would go away. Bailey was also on a very awful med at this time, causing out of control behaviors, depression, aggression, and again causing him to miss weeks of school.

Then he started the Ketogenic diet. A year later, he is not seizure free, but medicine free and paralysis free. He is still having many seizures a night, sometimes resulting in no sleep but he is 100% during the day. He has only missed two days of school due to epilepsy this year, and we are in the third quarter already! He is getting straight A's and had not one behavior issue!

The diet has improved his quality of life dramatically. I hope the success will continue. Only time will tell. But I will take what we have received for now. He is back to a happy nine year old boy who is able to get out of bed on his own two feet, and control the way he wants to behave throughout the day.

The Ketogenic diet has given him the best year he has had in a long time. I feel it is great success in Bailey's battle. For today we are steady. Nights bring hell and terror but he is able to function normally and happily on a daily basis. It has been the greatest year yet, in spite of the difficulty of the diet.
T. Anasenes, Chicago IL

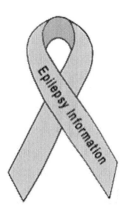

Women and Epilepsy

Everyone with epilepsy is at risk for bone density loss (BDL) due to antiepileptic medications. Post menopausal women have a greater risk. But the turnout doesn't have to be dismal. You can avoid all the complications by consuming enough calcium 1200 – 1800 mg. daily. It must be taken with vitamin D and separate from iron at 600 mg. intervals. (*You can only absorb 600 mg. at a time*). Do not put it off! Your bones won't put it off, so you shouldn't either.

Smoking, Alcohol, and Obesity

Smoking, alcohol, and obesity are all threats, and challenges for your body to consume and utilize calcium. So, if you're guilty of one or more, gain control over them now! They're already a risk to your body and certainly not worth broken bones, a hunched back, and a shorter body! Don't give the threats a helping hand at destroying your bones, as well as the possibility of causing seizure activity.

Maintaining healthy bones is no joking matter. You need to have a bone density scan to check for osteopenia (thinning of the bones) and osteoporosis (*reduction in bone mass*). You don't have to be 50 years old or over (menopausal) to be concerned about your bones.

When you have epilepsy, your concern starts after you take the first pill. So get concerned now, not scared, just concerned. Use your concern to stay on track with taking your calcium, and getting your bone density test (DEXA). See: *Tests*. The regularity for testing depends on the result of your last test or changes in your height.

If bone loss has already begun, calcium 1200 – 1800 mg. with vitamin D, separate from iron at 600 mg. intervals (*You can only absorb 600 mg. at a time*) is usually adequate to resolve the problem. Your doctor can help determine how much calcium is appropriate for you. Your doctor can also prescribe selective estrogen receptor modulators (SERMS), non-hormonal oral medication. They mimic estrogen's effects on bone with potential risks. Do not consider the short term hormone replacement therapy, pill or patch because they increase seizure activity.

Birth Control: You should be aware that some AEDs can interfere with the effectiveness of oral contraceptives so you should discuss this with your doctor. They may be able to prescribe a different kind of medication or suggest other ways such as an intrauterine device (I.U.D.) to avoid an unplanned pregnancy. It's very important to take responsibility to get educated and discuss it with your doctor.

If you're sexually active, *an unplanned pregnancy is possible even while on birth control.* Women who have the possibility to become pregnant should take folic acid during their childbearing years. With that in mind, you should take at least 400 mcg. folic acid (folate) daily. If you start taking a high dose of folic acid along with Dilantin or Phenytek you should have your blood levels checked regularly to see whether the folic acid is causing your medication levels to be lower than expected. Having a low blood level could increase the risk of seizures.

> ### *The following AEDs can cause a deficiency in folic acid by interference with absorption:*
> - Depakote
> - Dilantin
> - Tegretol (including XR)
> - Carbatrol, and
> - Phenobarbital

Pregnancy: Women who have epilepsy are quite capable of having babies considering there's no other condition thwarting the possibility. There is a 10 – 12% chance of inheriting epilepsy if the parent has epilepsy and the likelihood is more if the parent is the mother. However, the chance of inheritance drops if the onset of the mother's epilepsy was after age 35. Women who take anti-convulsant drugs need to plan their pregnancy carefully with the supervision of their epileptologist. If you're pregnant or planning to become pregnant, you should avoid taking high doses of vitamin D.

It's necessary to have your neurologist, epileptologist work closely with your gynecologist. The frequency of congenital birth defects have been recognized to increase two *to* three times as a result of the anti-convulsant medications causing, fetal anticonvulsant syndrome (FACS). But this doesn't mean your baby will surely have problems. The increased risk means approximately 5 – 10% of babies born to women taking anticonvulsants during pregnancy will have problems. But you can take part in preventing complications. Be sure to stay in close contact with both your gynecologist and epileptologist.

AEDs Connected to FACS:

- Tegretol (Carbamazepine)
- Phenobarbital (Phenobarbitone)
- Dilantin (Phenytoin)
- Carbatrol (Carbamazepine)
- Depakote (Sodium Valproate)

Take caution with new medications.

All the medications listed above are known to cause problems in babies who have been exposed to them during pregnancy. However, it is known that other anti-convulsant medications are safe. Therefore, if you are taking one of the medications proven to cause FACS, you can have your medication changed long before conceiving. To reduce the chances of FACS, be sure to take the recommended supplements of folic acid (400 mcgs.) which every women should take when trying to conceive and in early pregnancy. Folic acid cuts the chance in half and reduces the risk of some of the congenital problems seen in fetal anti-convulsant syndrome.

Be sure to take the recommended supplements before pregnancy. They are used in your body to make new cells. If you have enough folic acid in your body before you get pregnant as well as continuing throughout your pregnancy, it can help prevent all major birth defects.

Menopause: Menopause is defined as twelve continuous months without a menstrual cycle. Peri-menopause lasts for approximately five years before menopause and is a time when hormones change a lot. During menopause, levels of estrogen and progesterone fall dramatically because the ovaries stop functioning. This change in hormones may affect seizure control. With menopause, seizures may become less predictable. One study showed that if women had seizures linked with their menstrual cycle (catamenial epilepsy), they were more likely to have better seizure control after menopause. However, during the five years leading up to menopause (perimenopause), these women were likely to notice an increase in seizures.

Treatment Options for Menopausal Seizures:
- Adjustment of medication around expected time of seizures.
- Hormone therapy
- Surgery
- Vagus Nerve Stimulator

Catamenial Epilepsy

Catamenial epilepsy is triggered by hormones which influence seizure activity. Estrogen and progesterone affect the excitability of brain cells. Estrogen tends to excite them while progesterone calms them. During the course of your menstrual cycle, the hormone levels change in the blood. Approximately half the women with epilepsy during childbearing years report an increase in seizures related to their menstrual cycle. Seizures occurring predominantly during a particular time of the menstrual cycle are referred to as catamenial epilepsy. It is not a different condition with different types of seizures.

It simple defines the fact that seizures that occur around the following predictable times:

- Just before and/or at the onset of bleeding (day 1) due to a drop in progesterone.
- During the second half of the cycle (days 15 – 28) particularly in women with abnormal cycles.

Treatments for Catamenial Epilepsy

Women who suffer from catamenial epilepsy may benefit by taking hormone therapy. Hormone therapy is an alternative adjunctive therapy for women who have the tendency toward seizure activity and/or worsened seizures around the time of menstruation. When it comes to hormone therapy, it's important to take caution and review all the risks and benefits prior to considering this form of treatment.

Hormone Replacement Therapy (HRT)

A combination of estrogen and synthetic. Using progesterone has been found to relieve some women with complex partial seizures but estrogen can increase seizures. If you or your family has a history of breast cancer or a history of blood clots, you should not take hormone replacement therapy.

Possible side effects of estrogen and progesterone:
(Depend on length of treatment, dosage amount, and other medications)
- Anxiety
- Blood clots
- Breakthrough bleeding
- Breast cancer
- Depression
- Excessive hair growth or loss
- Fluid retention
- Heart problems
- Hot flashes
- Sleep disturbances
- Irregular menstrual period and discomfort

- Kidney problems
- Loss of sex drive
- Low blood sugar levels
- Migraine headaches
- Mood changes
- Vaginal dryness
- Weight gain
-

Possible benefits:
- Decreased seizure frequency
- Shorter seizure duration

Natural progesterone therapy, (bio-identical hormones) is derived from yams and is bio-identical to ovarian hormones. They function like those your body produces. The chemical structure matches the hormone it's replacing. The molecular structure of the hormones is indistinguishable from that of natural hormones produced in your body. Natural hormones are alternatives to synthetic hormones such as birth control pills. They are appealing because they work in a way in which your body can metabolize them as it was designed to do, minimizing side effects. Progesterone is an experimental potential treatment. Oral progesterone has a six to eight hour half-life in the bloodstream, so it's typically taken three times daily.

It's important to take the progesterone during your menstrual cycle. Generally, progesterone is typically begun on day 14 of a 28-day cycle to mimic the body's natural production. For example it's continued as 200 mgs. every eight hours, until the 28th day. The hormone is tapered by one pill per day until off, usually trailing two days into the next cycle. The reasoning for the specific hormone schedule is to keep the estrogen to progesterone ratio favorable, and to avoid causing progesterone withdrawal effects.

With the onset of menses, the new cycle starts as day one and the progesterone begins again on the next day 14. This two weeks on and two weeks off pattern is usually easy to adapt to and does not interfere with your natural cycle or prevent ovulation, like birth control pills. Natural hormone therapy has also successfully treated certain anxious, irritable forms of premenstrual syndrome (P.M.S.)

European medical studies suggest that bio-identical hormones are safer but haven't been studied long enough to determine their safety for women who had breast cancer or even a family history with breast cancer. It's up to you to do your homework!

Prometrium (brand name of a natural progesterone therapy) contains peanut oil and is obviously not appropriate for anyone allergic to peanuts. However, micronized progesterone capsules from a compounding pharmacy can be made using a different type of oil in order to replace the peanut oil.

It should *not* be used in combination with estrogen for the prevention of cardiovascular disease. It should be used for the shortest possible length of time at the lowest *effective* dose, to obtain the benefits and minimize the chance of serious side effects for long – term treatment. Consult your doctor or pharmacist for more details.

Possible side effects:
- Drowsiness
- Sudden numbness or weakness especially on one side of the body
- Fast or pounding heartbeat
- Chest pain or heavy feeling
- Dizziness
- Light – headedness
- Bloating
- Breast tenderness
-

Benefits:
- Decreases seizure activity.
- Doesn't inhibit estrogen's ability to raise good cholesterol.
- Micronized," chopped up" which makes it easier for the body to absorb.
- Shorter seizure duration.
- Taken orally but vaginal suppositories are available.

Risks:
- Fluid retention
- Glucose intolerance
- Depression

Diamox (acetazolamide) A mild diuretic considered to be a *sulfa* drug because of its chemical properties. It can be a possible adjunctive AED. For most women with epilepsy who have predictable menstrual cycles, Diamox is given a few days premenstrually. Your doctor will not prescribe this medication if your sodium or potassium levels are low, or if you have kidney or liver disease, including cirrhosis. Diamox should not be used in conjunction with aspirin. The effects if combined with aspirin can range from loss of appetite, sluggishness, and rapid breathing to unresponsiveness. The combination can be fatal.

Possible side effects:
- Change in taste
- Frequent urination
- Loss of appetite
- Dizziness
- Nausea
- Vomiting
- Ringing in ears
- Tingling in hands or feet

Benefits:
- Lessened seizure activity
- Reduction or complete seizure control

Risks:
- May increase risks of side effects for Tegretol
- Decreased calcium
- Bone marrow depression
- Birth defects (if taken while pregnant)

A True Story about a Woman's Attempt to Gain Control over Catamenial Epilepsy

I had just finished my first year of college, working as a part-time certified nursing assistant, and applied for nursing school. My health was great. I was almost three years seizure free! At my last appointment, the neurologist discussed when a good time would be for me to go off my medication. I knew at that time, it was definitely not a good time because school was going to get very stressful, especially if I was accepted into the nursing program. I loved my job working in home health. It really made me feel good to feel needed. It was also perfect for school. My client was amazing.

In December of 2007, after working a weekend with my client and taking finals the following week, I was exhausted. I had just driven to the gas station after work to fax in my time sheet and was talking to Mr. Bob, the owner, when I woke up in an ambulance. I had missed my medication the evening before. I was devastated! I think Mr. Bob was even more devastated. Ha ha! He had no idea what was happening. Poor guy! I knew exactly what had happened and it made me nauseous. My parents arrived and drove me to the hospital however we could not get in until morning. I just wanted to go to sleep, forever! The following day I was fine. I went back to work and took my finals the following week. However, I was not emotionally okay.

A seizure had never affected me this way before. I had my ups and downs in the past but this just came at a really bad time. I began to constantly worry about everything in my life. How would I get through nursing school? Would I ever be independent? Could I have children? All of the terrifying things I thought I had outgrown suddenly come back. I began having anxiety attacks, especially when I went out in public. The most difficult thing was giving up my driver's license for six months. I was so disappointed and stressed out. How was I going to continue school and my job without driving?

I wanted to give up. On top of it all, I had to find a new neurologist because mine had retired. I made an appointment with an epileptologist in the medical center in Houston but it would not be for another month. I wanted answers now! Meanwhile, I visited my general physician and told her what happened. She gave me something for the anxiety, which eventually went away, thank God! I also received the Depo-Provera shot for hormone suppression.

The seizures I had always occurred around, if not during, the time of my menstrual cycles. In a study I read, an option for treating catamenial epilepsy was Progesterone therapy. Progesterone is what the Depo-Provera shot contains. The purpose for the shot was to eventually stop my menstrual cycles, and possibly the seizures too.

The doctor went over some of the possible side-effects I would experience but not all. She said it could take up to a year for the shot to fully stop my cycles. The shot would last for three months and once I received it, there was no reversing it. Being an advocate of my own health, I should have researched more before making a decision. I guess I was desperate to try anything. I very soon regretted it. I was fine the first few weeks after the shot. I did not really notice any difference, not that I expected a single shot to cure me.

I began to get a little moody and down, however I was down before I got the shot. Then I did my research one night and really started to worry. There was nothing good that came from this shot other than it stopping your cycles. The side effects were terrifying and my doctor had not even mentioned most of them. Something told me this was not going to be good. I was preparing myself to go back to school, and the week before school began, I started feeling terrible. My cycle began as usual but had not stopped. I was aware of this, however not prepared for it.

My appetite was poor and getting worse. I was just not hungry, and I felt as if I was forcing myself to eat. Worst of all, I had no motivation to do anything. I could laid in bed all day and just sleep. I was very scared. I finally told my mother I needed help which I am sure she already suspected! My father and her both began taking off work to make sure I ate. However, I still had no appetite. I knew they were worried. I was also not sleeping well at night and terrified of having another seizure. School began the next week without me. I had no idea what to do or where to find an answer.

I went to work one day that week. I barely made it through my shift because I still could not eat. I had to do something! The next day I went to the hospital for severe dehydration. I was given some medication for nausea, and my blood tests revealed my medication was at a toxic level. The hospital referred me to a local neurologist. But the appointment would not be for almost another two months. I needed answers now! I needed food now! I called my boss and explained everything that was happening.

I really did not want to leave my client but my health came first. She understood greatly, at what made me feel better. I could go back to work when I felt healthy enough to do so. Then I decided what classes I really needed to take, as well as the ones I could do without right now. I knew if I took the semester off, I would feel even worse just sitting at home. I made an appointment to see the disabilities counselor at school and explained my situation. She got me into the classes I wanted. I felt better. But I needed something to get me through the next three months until the shot wore off. I went to another general physician the following week and explained my situation.

I had lost almost ten pounds and I looked horrible. The only good thing was I could fit into my clothes better. Ha ha! She prescribed some low dose anti-depressants to get my appetite back. It worked perfectly, thank God! I was so relieved! The bad thing was I could not sleep at night as a temporary side effect. I was prescribed a sleep aid. So here I am twenty years old and already taking three medications. Wow, not good! I kept reminding myself, it's only temporary. I also scheduled an appointment with a therapist to talk about anything that was bothering me. My family was more support than I needed but sometimes it is more comfortable talking to a complete stranger.

Slowly but surely things began to get better. My appetite returned, and I was getting out of bed every day. My grandparents drove me to school twice a week but other than that, I was a prisoner in my home! Ha ha! I found things to occupy my time that I had not done in so long. I enjoyed the time to myself a lot at times. I was very worried that I would be behind in school because I was not taking as many classes. However, I had taken as many classes as I could for nursing in the past year, so some time off would not hurt me. I welcomed the break with open arms and was very thankful.

Now that I look back on everything that happened during this time, although I did suffer a great deal, I believe it was all for good reason. I have lost nothing, and I have gained so much. I had not been to church in over six months, and I went for the first time about a month ago. I had never been so thankful. Just to be able to get out of bed and eat. Ha ha! Although I pray that I will never experience anything like this again, it has made me so much stronger in my faith. I believe that is exactly what it was, a test of my faith. I am currently attending school. I have switched my major from nursing, and although I have not found an answer yet, I thank God for giving me another day filled with hope.

A. Jewell, Santa Fe TX

More True Stories

I have lived with Epilepsy since the age of 12. I am about to turn 43. When they first figured out that I had epilepsy, the doctor back then told me that I would probably never drive or have children. At 12 years old that didn't sit well with me. I wanted to learn to drive. After years of getting my blood levels checked, seizures, and having to deal with people feeling sorry for me, that got on my last nerve.

I finally got to the point in my life where I wanted to have children. I went through a lot of tests and what not. The only way for me to have children was to take one of my medications away that may cause birth defects. Well of course I had some seizures. Then I finally got to the point where the seizures were controlled. I now have three children! I'm on my second and last marriage and I drive! I showed them! I have been seizure free for about nine years. I do still have those lovely auras from time to time but I do what I can to calm myself and they go away. The only thing that I have a problem with is that people think they know all about epilepsy but they really don't! Some will tell me they are sorry.

My response is "it is okay." It's a way of life for me! I have no choice but to live with the disorder. I really can't stand people that hold people with epilepsy back from succeeding in the job force. I deal with a lot of that stuff at my job. I experienced that last year but I got over it. I decided if they want to have the stress, they can have it. Now I am fine. I'm living my life the best that way I can each day. I am so very grateful for all my friends here on Myspace, that deal with the disorder also.

J. Nix, Knoxville TN

I was diagnosed with epilepsy when I was seven years old. My doctors expected me to grow out of it by puberty. But in junior high I started to have grand mal seizures. Through a few test runs with different medications (and a lot of awful side effects) it was finally under control. And then a year after high school they just disappeared. No more seizures! I was so grateful. I always wanted a family, and I was worried that while pregnant, I would fall into traffic one day and injure the baby. I actually have walked in front of cars before, so it wasn't that much of a long shot. But now I was seizure free, and my husband was coming back from the army. Needless to say, I got pregnant shortly after! I did have problems with the pregnancy even without having epilepsy.

I was diagnosed with toxemia and my son was born at 28 weeks. One of the side effects of toxemia is seizures, and with my preexisting seizure disorder my epilepsy is back. But I still feel blessed that I have a son who is in perfect health. If I have to live with epilepsy for the rest of my life, then bring it on! Now I have a beautiful son.
Y. Johnson, Denver CO

When Daniel was born, we didn't notice anything really out of the ordinary though he was quite a floppy baby. By the time he was crawling I was already pregnant with his sister. When it came to walking at first we thought he was just lazy. Then we started to get concerned when he still wasn't walking by 18 months. So I started taking him to physiotherapy. It turned out that he has a condition called hypotonia which basically means he is too flexible. He had speech and language therapy since he was 2 ½ years old because he had little speech and language skills.

Now he's five and has to go to a school which caters to his special needs. Daniel would not be able to cope in a mainstream school due to a number of reasons. He has difficulties with fine motor skills which mean he can't hold a pen to write, he struggles to use any kind of scissors, and cannot use a fork properly. His gross motor skills cause him to be very clumsy and hard to ride a bike. I can't remember the last time he wasn't covered in bruises from falling over. His speech makes it difficult to interact with teachers. He can't find the words which makes him very frustrated and angry.

Daniel still has to wear a nappy (diaper) at night because he has no control over his bladder. Although he doesn't wear a nappy during the day, he has very limited control over his bladder. He cannot dress himself because he gets everything mixed up and he can't button, zip, tie laces, etc. Another thing we have to deal with is he has no sense of danger at all. He would think nothing of just stepping into a road.

Daniel suffers with recurring infections mainly ear and chest. He was admitted to the hospital once due to a chest infection. He can get very emotional if he sees something sad on TV. He will get very upset. He doesn't like any changes to his daily routine and he can only follow one simple instruction at a time otherwise he won't understand. Daniel also has a developmental delay of about 15 months.

There is no medication for any of this. The best there is to offer is physiotherapy. My youngest child Jessica doesn't have it as bad as Daniel but she too, has problems. She has some difficulty with motor control. She is very clumsy and looks like she is going to fall over when she runs. She has speech and language problems but luckily she will be able to go to mainstream school. A speech and language therapist will be going to the school to have therapy sessions on a weekly basis. Jessica has bad temper tantrums. She has hit, punched, bit, kicked, and head butted me, her dad, and brothers. She is always seeking attention.

Like her brother, she has no sense of danger and would also walk out onto a main road. I have an older son who luckily enough avoided most of it. He only had one thing wrong. He had something called pyloric stenosis. He was operated on when he was six weeks old. He had no problems since. My two youngest, Jessica and Daniel both have facial features that go with FACS. They have a broad flat nasal bridge, thin top lip, narrow forehead, and tightly packed teeth.

We were never given any warnings that my medication could be harmful to my children. When I was pregnant with my two youngest children, I was on Epilim. I was on Tegretol with my oldest. We had to fight to get a proper diagnosis because most doctors hadn't even heard of it. We don't know what the future holds because we don't know how they will be affected as adults. We take each day at a time and deal with all the obstacles that come our way. They are great kids and couldn't imagine life without them. It can be hard at times but they are worth it!
T. McKay, Cheshire England

I'm a 25 year old mother of two girls and have epilepsy! I started having over 200 petit mal seizures daily in sixth grade. Within a year the grand mals came. The doctors said they weren't sure what caused them. Although I know my real dad has epilepsy. It took the doctors four years to get them somewhat controlled. I was a kid and didn't like taking the medication because the side effects were really bad. They caused my hair to fall out, and I gained 60 pounds. I just got tired of not remembering anything.

I was "Jessa with epilepsy" for many years and eventually realized I was Jessa, a *mother, daughter, and sister with epilepsy.* I have been able to teach my oldest daughter about epilepsy, what it is, what to do, and why it happens to mommy. By the time she was two she knew the last seizure tested her. She took care of me when she was only three and stayed by my side after she called 9-1-1.

It's been four and half years since my last seizure. They are controlled by my medication. Every day, I want to flush them and not have to take them but I know I have to! I only have seizures when I don't take my medication, and if I eat hot dogs or anything with MSG! Yes, it sounds crazy but it never fails.

I have struggled with epilepsy for many years. Friends don't want to worry whether or not their friend will fall and have a seizure. It does show who loves you though! It has made me a stronger person. I want there to be more awareness on the cost of seizure medication and help for someone who can't afford them which causes them to have a seizure. I have been there and it's the hardest thing I have been through. I had to choose between pills for the night or milk for my baby. This should not happen and there should be more help out there.

Jessa, Dayton OH

Jessa's yearning has been answered. See: *Patient Assistance Program and/or Discount Prescription Cards*

Appendix

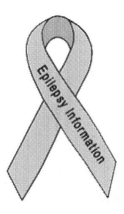

Patient Assistance Programs

As you are surely aware, medication can be so expensive without insurance that it can be almost impossible to purchase. If you're in a situation to choose between buying groceries or medication you need to review this chapter carefully.

If you work, you need to investigate whether or not your state provides medical assistance for workers with disabilities (M.A.W.D.) by contacting your local welfare office. Not all states provide this desperately needed program. Many had them at one point but in time were cut back or simply discontinued.

Reimbursement assistance is sometimes available for patients who have health insurance and need help securing appropriate coverage. Since help can be limited in your state or simply in your personal situation, you might be eligible for help to get your medication through a patient assistance program. Patient assistance programs are often available for certain individuals who are uninsured or have significantly limited health insurance. For another option See: *Discount Prescription Cards*

Brand Name Medication P.A.P. Provider

Ativan SCBN Select Care Benefits Network
(888) 331-1002 *Ask for Randall*

Banzel Eisai (855) 347 2448

Carbatrol XR Shire Pharmaceuticals (888) 227-3755

Depakene Abbvie Corp. (800) 222-6885

Depakote SCBN Select Care Benefits Network
(888) 331-1002 *Ask for Randall*

Diamox SCBN Select Care Benefits Network
(888) 331-1002 *Ask for Randall*

Diastat Valeant Pharmaceuticals International
(866) 268-7325

Dilantin Pfizer, Inc. (800) 707-8990

Felbatol Meda Pharmaceuticals (800) 593-7923

Frisium SCBN Select Care Benefits Network (877) 331-0362
Ask for Randall

Gabitril Cephalon Cares Foundation (877) 237-4881

Keppra UCB Pharmaceutical (866) 395-8366

Klonopin Rx Outreach Hope (800) 769-3880

Lamictal Glaxo Smith Kline (866) 728-4368 (*you must be pre-enrolled by an advocate*)

Lyrica Pfizer, Inc. (800) 707-8990

Mysoline Valeant Pharmaceuticals International
(866) 268-7325

Neurotin Pfizer, Inc. (800) 707-8990

Onfi Onfi Support Centre (855) 345-6634

Oxtellar SCBN Select Care Benefits Network
(877) 331-0362 A*sk for Randall*

Peganone Lundbeck Inc. (866) 209-7604

Phenobarbital SCBN Select Care Benefits Network
(877) 331-0362 A*sk for Randall*

Phenytek SCBN Select Care Benefits Network
(877) 331-0362 *Ask for Randall*

Potiga SCBN Select Care Benefits Network
(877) 331-0362 *Ask for Randall*

Sabril Lundbeck Inc. (866) 209-7604

Tegretol (XR) Novartis (800) 277-2254

Topamax Johnson and Johnson Patient Assistance Foundation
(800) 652-6227

Tranxene Lundbeck Inc. (866) 209-7604

Trileptal Novartis (800) 277-2254

Vimpat UCB Pharmaceutical (866) 395-8366

Zarontin Pfizer, Inc. (800) 707-8990

Zonegran Rx Outreach (800) 769-3880

༄

SCBN Direct you to patient assistance programs as well as additional availability.

RxAssist a.k.a. Xubex *Provides generic medications at affordable prices without long applications to fill out. However, there's no guarantee you'll get the same manufacturer every time. See: Medications and Possible Side Effects, Refer to: Generics Vs. Brand Name*

The representative companies and/or telephone numbers are subject to change. If you are non-eligible for a P.A.P., See: *Discount Prescription Cards*

Program Information

Please note the federal government provides the income poverty guidelines. Therefore, if you do not qualify for one company regarding your income you will probably not qualify for other companies.

Rarely companies determine their own income guidelines instead of using the federal government's. Although eligibility differs from program to program, they all have three universal criteria which include proof of income, lack of prescription insurance, and United States citizenship.

You may need the following information in order to qualify for a P.A.P.
- Notarized application
- Proof of income (income tax return (1040) or IRS verification)
- Provider centered programs filled out by both you and your doctor
- Verification for household persons
- Information necessary if ineligible for Medicaid or Medicare
- Doctor's written prescription

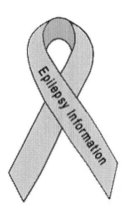

Epilepsy Information

Discount Prescription Cards

You have an option to gain access to immediate savings on hundreds of brand and generic prescription medications with unbelievable savings through stress free prescription discount cards! The cards are free and the medications can be up to 90% off! This seems too good to be true, but it is true! How is this possible? The discount card companies approached pharmaceutical companies and made a deal to lead *cash paying* customers to them in order that they honor the discount card! Apparently, it's appealing enough to contract thousands of pharmacy's to help under or uninsured patients.

Look for several sites that cover your medication(s). Print a card from each of them so they're available for price comparison at the pharmacy (prices and discounts may vary between pharmacies). You may also be able to use one of the cards to cover other medications! The cards are free. Print them off, and enjoy the savings!

Typical Universal Benefits:
- Everyone qualifies
- No card or membership fee
- Most cards provide instant activation
- No deductibles
- No hidden costs

- No claim forms
- Mail order options
- No pre-existing exclusions
- Unlimited usage
- No rebate forms
- Card holders are usually eligible with other prescription insurance
- No income restrictions
- No long applications
- Instant savings
- Customer service contact telephone numbers available
- Cover all family members (some include pets)

All insurance entities which include national health care, have their flaws. If you are not qualified for a P.A.P. and the insurer will not honor your doctor's prescription regarding the brand name, dosage amount, or pill amount per day; the issue can be resolved very easily by utilizing discount card offers. For instance, if your prescription is to take four pills daily yet the insurance plan will only cover three daily you can get the insurance to cover the maximum amount and the discount card for the additional pills. Simply have your doctor write two prescriptions. One in the format the insurer will cover, and a second for the uncovered amount which will be used with the discount card. You're basically taking the opportunity to fill the medication deficit by using your insurance and the discount card.

This is a perfectly legal avenue to get the medication your brain needs but the "overhead" doesn't understand or appreciate. Do what you must to get the medicine you need.

Card Information

Buycheapr.com No telephone number available

Coast 2 Coast Rx (800) 931-8872 coast2coastrx.com

County Rx Card (866) 561-1926 countyrxcard.com

Drug Card America (888) 299-5383
drugcardamerica.com

Easy Drug Card (877) 891-2198 easydrugcard.com

Familywize (800) 222-2818 familywize.org

Help Rx (877) 839-5689 helprx.info

HSA Rx Card (866) 561-1926 hsarxcard.com

Sun Association (866) 662-1351 sunassociation.org

Internet Drug Coupons (877) 321-6755 internetdrugcoupons.com

Mighty Savings (800) 776-0760 mightysavings.com

Needy Meds (978) 281-6666 needymeds.com

Paramount RX (800) 928-4501 paramountrx.com

Prescription coupon search (888) 412-0869 ext. 4
rxsavings4free.com (manufacturer brand name discount)

PS Card (888) 516-2535 pscard.com

Rx Free Card rxfreecard.com

Rx Savings Plus rxsavingsplus.com

Together Rx Access (800) 444-4106 togetherrxaccess.com

True Rx Savings (800) 886-8412 truerxsavings.com

Take Caution Purchasing
Medications On the Internet

If you'd like to purchase your medication from the internet take note
to the following information:

To protect yourself from victimization, you should not buy medication online that:

- Is linked through another website and is not registered individually on a search engine.
- Sells a medication without a prescription.
- Sell from sites which are not approved by the FDA.
- Require that you link to another web site to purchase the medication.
- Does not provide a phone number and/or address to answer your questions.

Take note: Some online pharmacies are perfectly legitimate however you need to take caution when you purchase your medication over the internet.

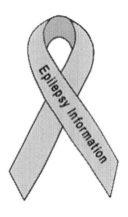

Websites and Resources

American Epilepsy Society Education Program aesnet.org

Americans with Disabilities Act (ADA)
A law that makes it illegal to discriminate against people with disabilities. The act applies to; employment, access to public places, and places of accommodation.
ada.gov

Anti epileptic Drug Pregnancy Registry
(888) AED-AED4 (233-2334)
aedpregnancyregistry.org

Assistive Technology Foundation
They will search their data base to find organizations that may be able to help you with your specific needs. (helmets, assistance dogs, etc.) To locate your local affiliate, search the foundation's name along with your state. (888) 744-1938

Canadian Epilepsy Alliance
(866) EPILEPSY (374-5377)
epilepsymatters.com

Charlie Foundation
Advocate for dietary therapy for epilepsy. Provide a wealth of information which includes ketogenic diet recipes, resources, supplies, and much more.
(310) 393-2347
charliefoundation.org
CharlieFoundationForum.org

Citizens United for Research in Epilepsy (CURE)
730 N. Franklin
Suite 404
Chicago IL 60610
(312) 255-1801
CUREepilepsy.org

Clinical Trials
Due to the fact trials are developed for different reasons, it's important to know what the researchers hope to learn before entering a clinical study/trial. Know the details expected of you prior to accepting the responsibility.
centerwatch.com
clinicaltrials.gov
neuropace.org

Daily Updates on Epilepsy Medical News
medicalnewstoday.com

Dandy-Walker Alliance, Inc.
4422 Clearbrook Lane
Kensington, MD 20895
(301) 919-2653
(877) DANDY WALKER (326-3992)
dandy-walker.org

E.E.O.C. Equal Employment Opportunities Act *(job protection)*
(800) 669-4000
eeoc.gov

Epilepsy.Com Well rounded website
Provides a personal ***epilepsy diary*** so you can document and print information for your records and doctor visits.

Epilepsy Action
epilepsy.org.uk

Epilepsy Advocate Information, insight, support, inspirational stories.
Epilepsyadvocate.com

Epilepsy Foundation
Search Epilepsy Foundation followed by your state.
epilepsyfoundation.org (National)

Epilepsy Magazines:

- ***Epilepsy USA***
epilepsyfoundation.org

- ***Epilepsy Advocate*** (free)
epilepsyadvocate.com

- ***Neurology Now*** (free)
neurologynow.com

Epileptologist Registry
epilepsyfoundation.org

Family Caregiver Alliance/National Center on Care Giving
(415) 434-3388
(800) 445-8106
caregiver.org

Human Relations Commission
(job protection)
Search "Human Relations Commission" along with your state.

International League Against Epilepsy
ilae-epilepsy.org

IRSA (International Radiosurgery Association)
(717) 260-9808
irsa.org

Ketogenic diet recipes
Pediatric advocate for dietary therapy
(310) 393-2347
charliefoundation.org

* Enhance your brain capacity *
lumosity.com

Make A Wish Foundation
(800) 722-WISH (9474)
wish.org

March of Dimes Foundation
1275 Mamaroneck Avenue
White Plains, NY 10605
(914) 428-7100
(888) MODIMES (663-4637)
marchofdimes.com

Mayo Clinic
mayoclinic.org

Medical Assistance for Workers with Disabilities (MAWD) search "Medical Assistance for Workers with Disabilities" along with your state to check for your state's availability.

National Association of Epilepsy
Find a comprehensive epilepsy center
naec-epilepsy.org

National Council on Patient Information and Education
(301) 656-8565
talkaboutrx.org

National Dissemination Center for Children with Disabilities
nichcy.org

National Organization for Rare Disorders (NORD)
P.O. Box 1968
55 Kenosia Avenue
Danbury, CT 06813-1968
(800) 999-NORD (6673)
rarediseases.org

Parents against Childhood Epilepsy (PACE)
(212) 665-PACE (7223)
paceusa.org

Project School Alert
Educate administrators, teachers, and students. Contact your local Epilepsy Foundation affiliate.
(800) 332-1000
epilepsyfoundation.org

Special Kids Network
(800) 986-4550
specialkidsnetwork.org

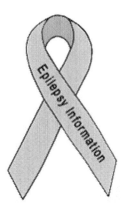

Glossary

Active ingredient Chemical part of a drug that works on the body to control or treat a condition or disease

Adjunctive therapy *a.k.a.* **add on therapy** Adding an extra medication to another medication presently taken to improve treatment quality.

Adverse event Side effect

Anoxia Lack of oxygen

Anticonvulsant Medication used to control or prevent seizures either acutely or chronically.

Antiepileptic Medication, procedure, diet or other substance used to prevent or stop seizures or convulsions.

Aphasia Defect in or loss of the ability to express oneself using speech, writing or signs; or to comprehend spoken or written language as a result of injury or disease of the brain's speech centers.

Apnea Stop breathing.

A-static (astatic) Inability to stand

Asymptomatic Without symptoms

Ataxia Inability to coordinate muscle movement caused by neurological impairment

Automatism Involuntary, undirected movement during complex partial seizures and atypical absence seizures

Benign Condition or disorder that is not harmful. It's likely to have a good outcome.

Bioavailability Amount of medication in a capsule or tablet that is actually metabolized.

Bioequivalence Equal performance of two or more substances used as therapy

Blood level monitoring Blood tests which check levels of antiepileptic drugs in your bloodstream. Blood samples are taken to ensure that a proper amount of the drug is being metabolized.

Breakthrough seizures Seizure's which occur despite drug therapy. Not controlled by standard medications and are also called refractory seizures.

Burr hole Relatively small opening made in the skull through a special drill used by a neurosurgeon.

Catheter Narrow tube made of elastic, rubber or plastic to pass through the body for evacuation or injecting fluids.

Cavernous angioma Abnormal tangle of blood vessels

Cerebellar Vermis Area between the two cerebral hemispheres

Cerebellum Posterior part of the brain responsible for coordinating voluntary muscle movements and maintaining balance

Cerebral cortex Outer region of the cerebrum, also called "gray matter" of the brain.

Cerebral hemisphere One of the two halves of the front part of the brain

Cerebrum Largest part of the brain responsible for voluntary muscular activity, vision, speech, taste, hearing, thought, memory, and many other functions.

Choroid Layers of blood vessels that nourish the back of the eye.

Chronic Affecting a person for a long period of time; a slowly progressing and continuing disorder.

Clinical trial *a.k.a.* **medical research/studies** Trials used to determine whether new medications or treatments are both safe and effective. One group of participants is given an experimental medication, while another group is given either a standard treatment for the condition or a placebo.

Clonic Involves muscle contractions and relaxations

Clustering Repeated seizures that follow immediately upon one another or which happen within hours of each other following periods without seizure activity

Cognition Process by which knowledge is acquired; awareness, thinking, learning and memory

Compounding pharmacy Creates custom formulations of drugs to your doctor's specifications

Congenital Present at birth.

Convulsion Involuntary contraction of the voluntary muscles common in generalized tonic-clonic seizures.

Convulsive Muscle movements like jerking or stiffening.

Corpus callosum Structure that links the two halves of the brain together, and permits them to communicate with each other

Cortex *a.k.a.* Cerebral cortex Thin outer layer of the brain which controls movement and the senses

Craniotomy Opening made into the skull for surgery to access the brain.

Cryptogenic Unknown or indeterminate origin

Dacrystic seizure "Crying" seizures.

Depth electrodes Thin wires placed deep in the brain to detect seizure activity that cannot be recorded from the surface of the brain.

Diagnosis Identification of an illness.

Disconnection syndrome Interruption of information transferred from one brain region to another.

Drop attack *a.k.a.* Atonic Sudden complete loss of muscle control and balance which results in collapse.

Dysarthria Speech that is characteristically slurred, slowed and difficult to understand. May have difficulty controlling the pitch, loudness, rhythm, and voice quality of their speech

Dyspraxia Partial loss of ability to perform coordinated movement

Efficacy Effectiveness of an AED in controlling seizures

Electrocorticogram Chart or record of the electrical activity of the brain by using electrodes in direct contact with it

Electrode Small, metal, cup-shaped disk attached to a wire.

Encephalitis Inflammation of the brain from an infection or as the result of other diseases; sometimes causes epilepsy.

Epilepsy Disorder of the nervous system with a pattern of repeated seizures. This is also termed seizure disorder.

Epileptic Having characteristics, related to, affected with epilepsy.

Epileptiform discharges Abnormal waves in an e.e.g. in patients with epilepsy that indicate signs of excitation in the brain.

Epileptogenic Cause an epileptic seizure

Epileptologist Neurologist who specializes in the care and treatment of epilepsy patients

Etiology The cause, study of the cause of a disease, or medical condition.

Excision "Cutting out," surgical removal

Frontal lobe Located in upper region of the head, behind the forehead. The frontal lobe controls decision-making, problem-solving or planning and motor movement.

Gamma knife "Knife-less" sophisticated computer technology which uses gamma rays to destroy targeted areas while sparing the surrounding tissue. Patients do not experience pain, and often may resume their usual lifestyle the day after treatment.

Gelastic seizures are called the "laughing seizure" because they may look like bouts of uncontrolled laughter or giggling.

Hemiclonic Similar to tonic-clonic seizure although only one side of the body is convulsive

Hemimegalencephaly Brain weight is greater than average for the age and sex of the infant or child

Hemisphere One half of the cerebrum. The largest part of the brain

Hydrocephalus Abnormal expansion within the brain that is caused by excess cerebrospinal fluid

Ictal Pertaining to, characterized by, or caused by an epileptic seizure.

Ictus Seizure or stroke

Idiopathic epilepsy Seizures for which there is no known cause; also called primary, inherited, genetic, or true epilepsy.

Incision To cut into. A cut made into an organ or tissue.

Infantile spasm The typical pattern occurs soon after awakening from sleep. It involves a sudden bending forward and stiffening of the body, arms, and legs. Arching of the torso can also be seen. They typically last for one to five seconds and occur in clusters, ranging from two to 100 spasms at a time.

Interictal Time period between seizures

Intractable Does not respond to treatment.

Investigational drug A drug available only for experimental purposes because its safety and effectiveness have not yet been proven

Ischemia Prolonged lack of blood supply to the brain

Kindling Brain "learns" to seize by seizing. A theory not all neurologists agree on.

Lateral Pertaining to the side.

Lateralize Localization of a function, such as speech, to the right or left side of the brain.

Lesionectomy Surgery to remove isolated brain lesions that are responsible for seizure activity

Lobe Section of the brain

Lobectomy Surgical removal of a lobe See: *Treatment Options*

Macrocrania Progressive unusually enlarged skull.

Mirroring Process where seizures start on only one side of the brain then in time "mirror" themselves on the other side of the brain causing an increase in the frequency of the seizures.

Mixed epilepsy Occurrence of several seizure types in the same patient.

Monotherapy Treatment with a single medication

Multifocal epilepsy Epilepsy in which the seizures come from a number of locations in the brain.

Myoclonic Single extensor movement of a limb; only infants have flexor myoclonic seizures.

Myoclonic astatic A seizure that involves a myoclonic seizure followed immediately by an atonic seizure.

Myoclonus Brief, rapid, shock-like jerking movement of a muscle or muscle group.

Narcolepsy Nonepileptic chronic ailment consisting of recurrent attacks of drowsiness and sleep; patient is unable to control spells of sleep but is easily awakened. Except for frequent sleep patterns e.e.g. is normal.

Neurologist Doctor who diagnoses and treats conditions of nervous system diseases and disorders

Neuropsychological testing Series of tests (written, oral, manipulation, etc.) designed to help understand where you are processing information in the brain.

Neuroradiologist Radiologist who specializes in the use of radioactive substances, X-rays and scanning devices for the diagnosis and treatment of diseases of the nervous system

Nocturnal seizures Occur during sleep

Non-convulsive Alterations of consciousness without jerking movements

Nonepileptic seizure Typically psychogenic in nature. Not of neurologic origin. Are not recognized on e.e.g. tests. May be due to temporary causes which include but not exclusive to; sudden drop in blood pressure, low blood sugar, high fever, drug or alcohol withdrawal, and medication side effects.

Noninvasive Not penetrating the body; as by incision or injection.

Nystagmus Rapid involuntary movement of the eyes

Occipital lobe Brain section/lobe at the rear of the head identified with vision.

Onset Beginning

Orifice Entrance or outlet

Paranoia Unfounded tendency to interpret the actions of other people as deliberately threatening or demeaning.

Paraxysmal Sudden outburst or eruption.

Paresthesias Sensation of prickling, tingling, or creeping on the skin.

Petit mal French term used in the 1800's to describe a small "spell" which is still used today to describe absence seizures.

Pharmacotherapy Medication therapy

Photic stimulation Stimulation of the brain by flashing light or alternating patterns of light and dark

Photosensitivity Reflex epilepsy; seizures are triggered by flashing lights or patterns (e.g., strobe lights, video games, or flipping and rolling of a television screen or computer). An estimated 3% of people with epilepsy are photosensitive.

Polymorph An organism that exists in different forms.

Polytherapy *a.k.a.* **polypharmacy** Two or more antiepileptic medications for seizure control

Postictal Period after a seizure which can last for minutes or days

Postictal confusion Temporary incoherence, inability to respond to contact or unfamiliarity with environment which commonly follows tonic-clonic, complex partial and atonic seizures.

Preictal Period prior to start of the seizure; sometimes called aura.

Prevalent Wide spread

Prodromal Indicating the onset of a seizure.

Progesterone Synthetic form of progesterone

Prognosis Prediction of the probable outcome

Pseudo seizure *a.k.a.* **Nonepileptic attack disorder** Sudden disruptive change in a person's behavior. It resembles epileptic seizures but has no electrophysiological changes in the brain. It may be related to physical illness, psychiatric disorder or emotional attacks.

Psychomotor retardation Generalized slowing of both physical and psychological activity.

Psychosocial Involving aspects of both social and psychological behavior.

Rapid clonic Spasms of muscle or group of muscles

Reflex epilepsy Rare epilepsy which occurs in response to specific sensory stimulus, including flickering light or patterns, sounds, tastes, smells, movements or sensations of touch.

Refractory Difficult to treat, unresponsive or of limited response to medication

Rescue medication Medication taken to prevent, reduce the severity of or stop a seizure while in action.

Resection Surgical removal of part of the brain

Seizure disorder Diagnosis used synonymously with epilepsy.

Seizure focus Area of the brain where the seizure begins.

Shunt Surgically implanted tube (catheter) placed in one of the fluid-filled chambers (ventricles) in the brain used to drain excess fluid and relieve pressure.

Spikes and waves Brain wave pattern on an e.e.g. during a seizure

Stenosis Constriction or narrowing of a passage or orifice.

Stereotactics Workstations designed to process and store digital data and images acquired by monitors, recorders, and/or imaging systems.

Subdural Area beneath the tough membrane (dura) which forms the outer envelope of the brain

Symptomatic With symptoms

Syncope Fainting due to a loss of blood flow to the brain; sometimes misdiagnosed as seizures.

Syndrome Set of symptoms characterizing a disease, disorder, or condition. See: *Children and Epilepsy*

Structural lesion Physical abnormality in the brain.

Temporal lobe Areas of the brain positioned at the side of the head behind the temples and which are involved in hearing, memory, emotion, language, illusions, tastes, and smells.

Teratogenic Medication or treatment with the potential to cause birth defects

Therapeutic Care provided to improve a condition; especially medical procedures or applications that are intended to relieve illness or injury.

Therapeutic range Range of medication levels in which most patients will experience significant therapeutic effect without an undesirable degree of adverse reactions. It's only used as a guide since; patients often require more or less medication for seizure control than suggested by the laboratory report.

Todd's paralysis Weakness after a seizure; originally used to describe muscle weakness on the side of the body opposite the side in which the seizure occurs.

Toxicity Occurs when a person has accumulated too much medication in their bloodstream, leading to adverse effects within the body. It may be caused when the medication dose is too high for the liver or the kidney is unable to remove the medication from the bloodstream; allowing it to accumulate in the body.

Transcranial magnetic stimulation Experimental procedure that exposes the brain to a strong magnetic field as a potential treatment for epilepsy

Transection Shallow cuts

Trigger Initial event that causes a seizure to take place.

Unilateral Affecting only one side

Vagus nerve Nerve which begins at the brain stem passes through the cranial cavity past the jugular, to the throat, larynx, lungs, heart, esophagus, stomach, and abdomen.

Ventricles Hollow cavities in the brain filled with cerebral fluid.

Vertigo Spinning sensation

Unacceptable Terminology
Amongst Our Epilepsy Friends

Disease *Epilepsy is NOT a disease!* It's a neurological disorder. A disease is chronically progressive and impairs normal functioning as a consequence of infection, inherent weakness, or environmental stress and can affect the entire body. However neurological disorders only affect the arrangement of the nervous system, causing confusion in the nervous system.

Epileptic The word "epileptic" should not be used to describe someone who has epilepsy because it defines a person by one trait. When you say you're epileptic that gives an image in a persons mind of a seizure. That's typically what they'll connect you with. They don't think about anything else like, you as a person, your family, your education or job, etc. In other words, when you say you're epileptic you're practically holding up a sign stating "Seizures define who I am."

A label is powerful and can create a limiting and negative stereotype. It is better to refer to someone as a person with epilepsy. If you want to share with others that you have epilepsy, simply say, "I have epilepsy." When you say you have something, it differentiates what you *have* from who you *are*. Keep in mind, if you are the person with epilepsy, and you don't mind using the word epileptic to describe your condition, you're teaching other people that it's okay to label the rest of us. Help us win the battle to be respected.

As an epilepsy advocate, I'm very active in my small community. Most people know me and that I have epilepsy. I'm far from embarrassed to talk about my condition. I use the information I learned through my personal experience to educate and help others. However, I chose to get away from the "looks" and bias of *how* people see *me*. People surpass seeing me as an epileptic because that's not how I introduce myself or represent who I am. They see me as a person who happens to have seizures and thrives on life. I'm not a seizure to them. I'm a *person* who's making a difference. I hope I'm getting my point across.

Fit Usually viewed as a "bratty" action. For personal comments by other epilepsy patients. See: *A Different Look at Epilepsy*. Refer to: *Terminology on a Personal Level*.

Illness Epilepsy is a condition, not an illness or disease.

My epilepsy, **my** seizures The word my suggests you "own" the epilepsy or seizures. You don't own them, you have them. It does make a difference how you word what you say. Instead of saying, my seizures or my epilepsy simply remove the word my or substitute it with the word the. Review the difference. "I only have my seizures when I'm sleeping." or "I only have seizures when I'm sleeping." As you can see you haven't changed the content or purpose of the sentence. "My epilepsy started when I was a teenager." or "I got epilepsy when I was a teenager." It'll take some getting used to as it did for me but it does make a difference, a huge difference.

Sufferer Suggests helplessness.

Victim Someone who is harmed by or made to suffer by an act.

If you're uncomfortable saying you have epilepsy, just say you have a neurological condition. You don't have to announce your condition. You don't owe it to anyone. Go with what you're comfortable with.

Terminology Breakdown

The following prefixes and suffixes are more likely to be used in the world of epilepsy. Attempt to learn the prefixes (beginning of the word) and suffixes (end of the word) If you come across words "on the spot" that are in a "different language" you will be able to decipher the word to at least have a basic understanding of its meaning. Learning terminology provides you with a great advantage to understand the mumbo jumbo of medical language!

Prefixes:

- **a, an** no, not
- **cephal** head
- **cerebr** brain, cerebrum
- **crani** skull
- **epi** above
- **neuro** nervous system
- **path** disease
- **peri** surrounding
- **post** after
- **pre** before
- **tonic** stimulating

Suffixes:

- **algia** pain
- **clonic** rapidly alternating muscular contracting and relaxing
- **ectomy** surgical removal of part or all
- **ic** pertaining to
- **itis** inflamation
- **lobo** section
- **ology** process of study
- **oma** tumor, mass
- **osis** abnormal condition
- **ostomy** creating a new opening
- **otomy** cutting into

Prescription Breakdown

- **bid** twice daily
- **tid** three times daily
- **qid** four times daily
- **po** by mouth
- **prn** as needed
- **dx** diagnosis
- **qhs** at bedtime
- **qd** once a day

"Initially" Important!

- **AED** antiepileptic drug
- **AEEG** ambulatory e.e.g.
- **CNS** central nervous system
- **DBS** deep brain stimulator
- **DX** diagnosis
- **ECU** epilepsy care unit
- **EEG** electroencephalogram
- **EcoG** electrocorticogram
- **GM** grand mal
- **GTC** generalized tonic-clonic
- **ICU** intensive care unit
- **IEP** individual educational plan
- **IV** intravenous
- **JME** juvenile-onset myoclonic epilepsy
- **MRI** magnetic resonance imaging
- **MSG** monosodium glutamate
- **NES** non-epileptic seizure
- **PET** positron emission tomography
- **RTL** right temporal lobe
- **TLE** temporal lobe epilepsy
- **VEEG** video electroencephalogram
- **VNS** vagus nerve stimulator

CEN
C.1

Made in the USA
Lexington, KY
12 August 2014